WHAT?!

A Fibromyalgia Survivor's Guide for Women

BETH McCAIN

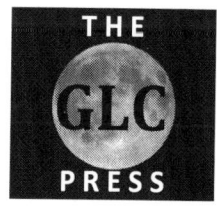

contents

WHY ME?	7
PHARMACOPIA	23
GETTING THROUGH TODAY	51
NO PAIN NO GAIN — *OH REALLY?!*	95
DON'T TAKE THIS LYING DOWN	109
YOU HAVE TO THINK OF YOU	133
POSITIVE THINKING	149
HELPING YOUR BODY AND MIND	155

CHAPTER ONE

Why Me?

You've picked up this book for myriad reasons. Maybe you suspect you might indeed have the condition known as Fibromyalgia or perhaps someone you know has it and you want to learn how to support them. Maybe the scientist in you wanted to read about something so strange, weird, and so totally debilitating that curiosity got the better of you, and here you are. Whatever your reason, you will find my take on Fibromyalgia a bit different than most. In this book you will discover what methods I have tried and used to mitigate Fibromyalgia as much as possible, and more to the point, what has actually worked.

You will also experience what it feels like to have this condition through a little bit of humor, because if I didn't laugh, I'd have to cry. I have had this crazy condition for most of my life but wasn't diagnosed until recently and now it all makes sense. Well, as much sense as you can make out of a condition that leaves no stone unturned in your body.

This isn't meant to demean this mysterious disorder that affects from three to six percent of the population, most being women. There is probably more than that, but because of the medical community's hesitance to even acknowledge this syndrome it will likely be a long time before we really know what the true numbers are.

Not everyone who has this condition sees the doctor whether from lack of insurance or just not wanting to deal with it by ignoring it. Fibromyalgia doesn't just go away. It takes a change in lifestyle but it can be a good change. Life *can* actually be better than it was before.

I've chosen to deal with it through humor and positive thought. You have to when every single patient's symptoms vary. No two Fibro Friends are alike. And just when you think you have it all under control, up pops another fibro symptom. I'm beginning to wonder if fibro is some kind of gypsy curse from generations past and it landed on me.

"I curse your family! No wait, I have a better idea. I curse your great-great granddaughter with a stupid condition that makes her want to gnaw her foot off."

Well guess what, Brunhilda, it worked!

Who named it, anyway?

Yes I know what Fibromyalgia stands for. It is from the Latin; fibro meaning fibrous tissue, myo meaning muscle, and algos meaning pain. Fibromyalgia has many different faces. It could have ended up with a much longer title.

It could have been called the muscle pain, joint pain, tendon pain, stiffness, aching, stabbing pain, hot fire feet, tender points, irritable bowel, incontinence, muscle spasms, depressive, shaking, coughing, extreme fatigue, brain fog, confused, loss of memory, cold like symptoms, vision problems syndrome. So guess I won't complain. They call it FM for short. Maybe that's because, like FM radio, you can hear it twenty-four hours a day. Why couldn't they have named it something much easier for all of us to pronounce? You know something like 'Feel Like a Butt' syndrome, or FLAB. That would work.

You go to your doctor and he listens as you describe your multiple symptoms and he says, "Do you feel like a butt?" And you say, "Why, yes, I do." "Well then," he concludes, "you have FLAB." That about sums it up.

This book isn't meant to give you all of the answers because quite honestly nobody has them. But will tell you what has worked for me. It is meant to let you know that you have someone who understands what you are going through who is also weaving her way through the wonderful world of Fibromyalgia.

Despite the many doctors out there who don't accept Fibro as a true condition, there are just as many who do recognize and respect this very real illness.

I am by no means diagnosing or telling you what to do. I am not a doctor. But I am letting you know what has worked for me, and that is a start. For all I know it could all change tomorrow because as you already know, that is exactly how Fibro spins its wicked web. It keeps you on your toes (while sending shooting pains to said toes), and messes with your physical as well as your mental state.

There is much speculation about what Fibromyalgia actually is. We do know that FM is a condition that is in the chronic pain category. This chronic pain is markedly amplified compared to persons who are not afflicted with FM.

It's possible that the neurological and hormonal and chemical changes of FM patients don't behave like those of most people and this causes our senses to be on high alert resulting in pain and the many other symptoms.

Our neuroendocrine systems process differently and our central nervous system says we are in pain even when slightly touched.

Two and two makes five.

"I can't quite put my finger on it but I just don't feel... *right.*"

This was my mantra for quite some time. Just when you think you may have cracked the code, here comes another medical test that says: You are A—OK! You are as healthy as a horse.

Doctors look at you sideways wondering what could possibly be bothering you. "Are you under a little stress?" they ask with a straight face.

"Uh... *YEAH!* I'm exhausted."

And I'm not talking about the kind that feels good after that wonderful five mile run. It's a kind of exhaustion that builds through the day. Not 'sleepy exhausted'. It's the "There is no way I could ever feel this tired in my life!" exhausted.

I am in pain.

I'm dizzy.

My muscles are twitching.

And still you don't believe me. Something is taking over my body, Doc, and you can't seem to find it.

"Here are some pills," the M.D. smiles with the lightest touch of condescension; "they might help you."

You are handed a prescription for an illness that they don't even recognize or acknowledge, but they figure the pills will get you to pipe down and let them take care of patients who really have something.

So I thought it best if I do a little self-diagnosis on the side. What could it hurt? Maybe I have Multiple Sclerosis or Lupus, perhaps. The more I searched the Web, the more convinced I became that I had millions of diseases. Each one described exactly how I felt. I picked up the phone.

"Hello? Yes, this is Beth McCain again. I was looking on the net... Can I hold? Sure."

You have no idea how many elevator songs there actually are until you're put on hold at my doctor's office.

"This is the nurse. You think you might have Multiple Sclerosis?"

"Well I was on the Net and..."

"Ms. McCain. Are the pills working?"

"I didn't take them."

"Why not?"

"Because you don't know what is wrong with me."

"Please hold."

"We've only just begun... to live... white lace and promises... a kiss for luck and we're —"

I was beginning to feel as if it was all made up. That's how they were making me feel. Now why would I make this up, I thought. Why would I play this cruel joke on myself?

" . . . Tall and tan and young and lovely, the girl from Ipanema goes walking, and when she passes, each one she passes goes — aaahhh . . . "

It's a cinch that the girl from Ipanema didn't have Fibro. The nurse came back on the line.

"Take the pills, Ms. McCain, and then we'll talk."

"Actually do you think the doctor could refer me to a neurologist?"

Deadpan voice.

"What for?"

"I'm dizzy and lights freak my eyes out. Maybe there's something going on in there."

I was grabbing at straws. I wasn't a doctor but I had to be since my own doctor wouldn't even acknowledge how I felt.

"I don't think..." she started.

"That's the problem. You don't think. I'm not making this up. I feel like crap. I would like a referral to someone who will take this seriously."

"It's not that we're not taking..." I cut her off.

"Referral, please."

"Hold on."

Back to the Girl from Ipanema for another two minutes

"It has to be approved."

"I can wait."

Two days later I got the approval to see a neurologist and that's where I first found some light at the end of the tunnel. (But even that light freaked my eyes out.)

Visiting the neurologist.

I was actually a little nervous as I filled out my paperwork. Was this the answer? I had been asking the Universe for some kind of answer for a very long time. I practice positive thought and it has helped me through many a problem over my lifetime.

I knew there was an answer and I had decided that I was not going to leave any stone unturned until I found out what was wrong with me. There was some kind of purpose in all this even though for the life of me I couldn't yet see why. But I trusted finding the answer. There was an answer and I hoped that it would be found here.

I wondered how I could advise helping your own health through positive thinking when I was experiencing such pain myself. I was advising others to visit their doctors but to make sure to visualize being well. It was then I began to understand that maybe this Fibro thing may help someone else. That's when I stopped fighting and avoiding how I felt and embarked on a journey to finding the physical me that I once was.

I knew that there was a purpose somewhere and starting with another new doctor might reveal it to be a large part of the answer.

I stepped into the examination room. I had printed out three pages of symptoms so I wouldn't have to repeat it once again to another doctor. I didn't care what they did to me even if it took probing my brain with science fiction robots to find the problem.

I sat down and then stood up. I paced back and forth and for a split second even thought about leaving. I sat in the corner and my husband watched me. Finally he said, "This isn't like you, Babe."

I rolled my eyes. "Oh, really?"

I was having a particularly hard day and it was reflected by my mood and the pain in my joints.

"I haven't been me for three weeks now."

This was the strange thing about this disorder. One day you feel great, the next day you can't walk. Five minutes later you can run a marathon and the next minute you're crawling across the floor to get to that much needed chocolate you're craving. I wish chocolate was the cure all. Why couldn't chocolate be the answer? I would eat it twenty-four-seven and feel better and better. Why not? Wouldn't it be great to actually learn that something they say is so bad for you is the cure? Hey, it could happen!

Round and round I'd go, over and over again, trying to find answers. No rhyme, no reason. I patted my husband.

"Sorry."

At least I had my wits about me. I breathed in and out and sat down waiting once again for another doctor. And then she came in.

I'd like to say that I heard angel's singing or saw an aura of white around her but I didn't. I was sitting there ready for another round of "Let's guess what Beth is experiencing?"

At first it started like all the others.

"You sure have a long list of ongoing symptoms here."

(Snicker from doctor.)

"I don't know what to tell you."

(She didn't know where to begin.)

"All your tests have come back normal."

She pored over my three-inch-thick pile of doctor's notes from all of the specialists I had been seeing while trying to chase down what I had.

She circled certain symptoms and then took off her glasses.

"What is it that you want to hear?"

No one had asked me that before. I thought for a moment and then began to cry from relief. She was *listening*.

"I just want a diagnosis. I want to be told that this is something that is physical and not just brushed off that it's stress."

She looked me over. "What do you do for a living?"

"I'm a positive thought author and speaker."

She laughed aloud. "You're a positive thought author? How are you staying positive through all this?"

My husband interrupted. "She does, even through her tears." My heart swelled as I fell in love with him again. He had my pain-filled back.

She rattled off some tests they would be doing. "We're going to connect you to some probes that will read your brain activity and we are also going to rule out Lupus. We're going to check your muscles and a few other things. Are you up for that?" I nodded, knowing that it didn't matter as long as there was the possibility of an answer.

"Could you hop up on the table please?"

"She can't hop anymore," my husband grinned. I walked over and did my best to get up on the table. She checked my reflexes and found that I couldn't extend my foot.

"Anyone ever check this?"

"Nope," I said. My confidence was rising. Finally someone checked something that hurt. She checked my elbows, neck, and knees. I jumped through the roof.

"I barely touched you. Has anyone checked this before?" She had a look in her eye like she actually might know what was going on.

I smiled. "No, but it hurts."

"So I think I know what's wrong with you."

That is when the angel chorus went into high gear. Someone might have an answer? She believes me!!

"I think you have Fibromyalgia."

She took my symptom checklist and ticked them off.

"Let's do the testing for all the things it could be and then we'll say for sure."

I went in for my brain wave test which really wasn't a bad experience. They put gel in my hair and placed probes on my sleep deprived head to read the rhythm of my brain. I fell asleep on the table and even got a nice new hairdo—gel and all—out of the deal. We went back to her office.

"Everything looks pretty normal. You do have an unusual rhythm to the brain but that's not really a problem."

"Okay! That explains it," my husband teased.

"So I'm going to give you what you want. Here's a diagnosis . . ."

What I'd been waiting for was about to happen. Someone understood, someone believes me, someone is going to make it all go away.

"You have Fibromyalgia. It isn't curable at the moment. We can only treat the symptoms. It's not life threatening even though it feels that way. It's possible that it is located in the central nervous system. Your body is saying that it is in pain when it isn't supposed to but still we're not quite sure why it happens.

"There are many theories as to what causes Fibromyalgia and what it actually is. We're researching and trying to figure out what it is but it's all speculation right now. Some don't believe that it's even a disorder but we're finding that it's a real physical condition.

"It's considered a syndrome because there are only symptoms involved. I believe it will be considered a disease not too far down the road.

Not every FM patient has the same symptoms. Some have just a few that are a mild annoyance, and some have more severe ones like you have.

"There are some things you can do but it's really going to be trial and error since every patient with FM is different. So let's start with this."

She handed me a prescription.

"YAY! I have something. It isn't all in my mind. I mean . . . what? Not curable? Don't really know why it happens? Only speculation? No miracle pill?"

So I got what I wanted, a diagnosis. I had fibromyalgia. I had the sniffing, sneezing, coughing, aching so you can't rest disorder and you wouldn't believe what I was going to have to do in order to get my life back. It was like an animal, sometimes predictable and sometimes unpredictable, but you are always on the alert just in case it decides to bite.

CHAPTER TWO

Pharmacopia

Like a wild animal, you have to learn what it loves and doesn't love and perform certain workarounds in order to get it to behave. Sometimes it makes no sense at all. You will have done everything you have always done (and then some) and the beastie brings out its pesky little Fibro knives and begins stabbing at you: *"Hey today I think I'll work on your temperature. So let's begin."*

Your face becomes flush right from beneath the skin and your husband even thinks that maybe you might be in the mood. But then two seconds later you have a creeping cold feeling that takes away the heat and makes you feel as if your neck and feet are buried in the Arctic tundra.

It can't be the whole body, just the neck and feet. A scarf on the neck later, and a pair of slippers on the heat-pain-sensitive-feet, and a pair of underwear (nothing else) and you're good to go. Underwear (for modesty of course) but cool enough for those spots that are on fire.

So how do I take care of it all? How do I continue to perform this job that I love with all of these little imps gnawing on my body? Through trial and error and just plain listening to what my body is trying to say. I then do my best to find something that will take care of certain symptoms.

I start with regular herbal concoctions, supplements, and homeopathy and then mix in the least amount of prescription medicine possible. I've tried what doctors say *won't* work and I've tried what they say *will* work. As you know we are each different, thus Fibro attacks patients differently. I've read book after book telling me what will not work and what will.

"Don't use herbal supplements" say many doctors. "They are useless." Tell my husband that when I fail to take an herbal supplement. He sees the difference *and I feel the difference.*

This doesn't mean that you randomly try every single thing that claims to cure Fibro because at the moment it isn't curable; but, what can be done is to lessen the symptoms. And try to remember that it isn't just 'in your head' should a product work for you that's been deemed worthless. Just do your research and listen to others who are veterans of this disorder. Listen to your doctor, listen to your body, semi-listen to what others have done, and find the answer. You don't have to suffer every day. You can lessen the pain and the annoying symptoms.

Part of my brand of Fibro is being extremely sensitive to any and all prescriptions or natural remedies. I always start out with half the recommended dose and then slowly raise the amount. Whatever works is what I stop at—never beyond the original dose and usually way under the suggested amount.

So what's been working for me?

I take loads of supplements. I can't wait for the day that I go to the store and find the gallon-size pill holders because that's the one I'll buy! What I take depends on the week and the ever-changing symptoms, but here's a list of what keeps me moving.

Baclofen

It is relatively inexpensive and it takes care of the muscle twitching and spasms during the day and at night. This is a prescription medication and is used for Multiple Sclerosis and spinal cord injuries. It's a muscle spasm medication.

My dose varies from week to week. It can be a little rocky when you start Baclofen but it is worth sticking it out. When I put the first dose in my mouth I began to feel worse. More tired (how's that possible; to feel even more fatigued?) and lethargic.

I felt like a walking noodle.

No brain and no brawn but after my system got used to it I no longer had the lethargic feeling and could think clearly with less pain. It immediately changed my restless night to one of calm void of any of the annoying twitching. I used to wake up at night watching my legs spasm to the rhythm of the Bobby McFerrin song, *Don't Worry Be Happy.*

They felt like one of those musical pipe organs that play of its own accord, but with

Baclofen the spasms are kept to a minimum. It even helped the profuse sweating I had been experiencing at night. I used to wake up every night at 3 a.m. with my face flush, kicking off my socks, then the twitching would begin but Baclofen has kept that at bay. No more nights of trying to figure out what shapes are in the ceiling. I snooze like a baby now. Every once in a great while I'll have a night where I can't sleep but that is usually due to the big bowl of ice cream I ate right before bed.

Black Cohosh Complex

I've had Fibro for a major portion of my life. It decided to really get going when I had surgery to have my ovaries removed. My uterus had already been taken soon after the birth of my youngest child, but I had not felt quite right since then. I began going to doctors to figure out what was going on and they found a mass on my ovary. They couldn't tell what it was so they decided the best course of action would be to go in and take a look. They thought I possibly had a cancerous tumor but when they got inside it turned out to be scar adhesions from the previous surgery and they brought in a gastroenterologist to remove the intestinal scars. Disgusting, yes, but we thought for sure this would take care of all my problems and any symptoms.

I was in euphoric bliss for six weeks after surgery. I healed nicely and hadn't experienced a single symptom. I slowly began walking around and thought, "This is it! It's all over!" But Fibro was just hiding, waiting for the perfect moment to come knocking at the door like an unwelcome house guest.

One night I woke up in the middle of the night with a spasm.

"Knock, knock. Anyone home?"

I rolled over and said, *"No. No one's home. They took you out."* And then, as each night came, I spent more and more time with my buddy, Fibro, and realized it was far from over. So now I had a grand scar *and* the symptoms.

At the six-week mark things began to get ugly. At the time I didn't realize that I had Fibro, but to read about it now I saw that I'm the classic fibromyalgic. A trauma of any kind (surgery, anyone?!) can trigger the symptoms full force.

Adrenaline from the surgery kept things at bay, and then as that calmed down Mister Fibro showed up and grabbed hold once again.

Reading on the internet, I found that women who have gone through menopause have the most severe Fibromyalgia and my body had just been thrown into menopause. Early. Go figure!

So I began the journey of menopause as well. And I've done my best to be vocal about what I take in prescription medicine. I prefer to take the lowest dose possible and then work my way up if need be but I will go with a teeny dose and see what I can possible take naturally that will help as well. In my perfect world I'd like to be off all medications but until then I do what I can to find the natural way and use the medications the doctor prescribes as the supplement.

That being said, make sure you have everything checked out before you think you may have FM. When the doctor asks you to take sleep studies, MRIs, estrogen levels, blood work, etc. Do what they ask.

Every little test you take will either rule out something or show you have something in addition to FM and they may have a way to ease your pain because of a separate diagnosis which in the long run helps your FM. Taking a sleep disorder study can reveal sleep apnea or seizures and if you do have one of these conditions it will only help to treat it.

There is a point where you have to say, " Enough is enough" but know that moment yourself. If your doctor seemed to be grabbing for straws because he/she doesn't want to admit you have FM (there are those doctors) then it's time to change to another one that understands and will work with you. You ultimate have the decision. It is your body...

I began to tell the difference between hot flashes and Fibro flashes hoping I could at least find something to quell the hot flashes. I found Black Cohosh and it worked; not only for my hot flashes, but for all of the other moodiness attached to the change of life. Black Cohosh is an herbal supplement that is known to help with menopause. It also has anti-inflammatory attributes as well as serving as a muscle relaxant. It is also available over the counter.

I continue to take it because, well, for lack of a better word, I'm a witch without it.

I tried going off it for a few days and my family basically held an intervention me.

"What have you stopped taking?" they cried. Obviously I'm notorious for doing that. Something works well and I try to back it off just in case the ol' body has decided to kick in.

"What are you talking about?" I asked, as my head spun around like Linda Blair in *The Exorcist.*

"You're off the Cohosh, aren't you?"

"Why, whatever do you mean?" I said with all the sincerity I could muster.

"Show me the box."

They had me. I had thrown out the empty box. No evidence that I was taking the Cohosh. I went down that day and picked up the Complex. Black Cohosh helps some of the symptoms whether they are hormonal or not. My mood is much better and so are the sweats. My muscles thanked me.

The Black Cohosh Complex comes in a day and night supplement. You take a pill in the morning and one at night. They contain all natural ingredients including Ginseng and Green Tea and of course the 'Witch be Gone' ingredient itself, Black Cohosh.

Estradiol Patch

Hot flash after hot flash and I couldn't figure out if it was Fibro or menopause. Many of us have estrogen issues and sometimes I wonder why they don't check for that first with women. I've always had 'female' problems when it became that time of the month. And the FM always flared during those days but now that I have been thrown into menopause it became a whole different ball game.

The Estradiol Patch has done a couple of things for me. Between the Black Cohosh and the patch I have now been able to sleep without the night sweating and my hot flashes are now at a minimum. Sleep is so important for anyone but is even more important to us FM patients. Sleep is the time for our bodies to rest and heal.

If you have ever had a hot flash, you know what I'm talking about. I had someone once say, "So you get hot...big deal." Yeah...you feeling like you're burning from the inside out and you just can't get cool. You sweat profusely and you feel as if it isn't your own body and then the agitation begins. The Fibro decides that this would be a good time to flare and then you get into the cycle of menopause and Fibro. It's like they feed off one another.

The patch and the Black Cohosh Complex took those symptoms and made them less and if you have Fibromyalgia anything to feel more normal helps... *Anything...*

Again, I am on one of the lowest doses possible. The patch has shown that there is less risk for any kind of cancer down the road opposed to the creams and prescription hormones.

It is all about your quality of life. If you are against taking anything and you are suffering, ask yourself, "How is my quality of life? If taking supplements and a few prescriptions will make my life 'feel' better, then your quality of life will be better.

Vitamin D

One of the severest symptoms of Fibro can be depression. It's true what they say about depression hurting not only you, but everyone around you. Imagine being a positive thought author while wrangling with bouts of melancholy. It has nothing to do with what I believe or who I am, it's just another little slice of the Fibro Pizza.

We get a lot of rain where we live and the rain can trigger seasonal mood disorder in some people. And since us Fibro patients feel worse on a physical level in the wintertime, it's no wonder that it rears its ugly head as depression.

So what's the fix?

There are a couple of things that help me. No matter what the weather is doing outside, I get out. I will sit with my umbrella on the porch and watch the clouds go by. Just getting out and breathing in the fresh air makes a significant difference.

With Fibro it always comes back to the little things you can do for yourself that give you the sanity. Sometimes we're unable to open a simple jar and other times we can hardly walk across the room. But taking in some of the fresh air outside is a must.

It's a must to have that time to yourself and to make sure you see the outside. Vitamin D is something that everyone who lives in a rainy or snowy area should take. Nothing replaces the sun but Vitamin D provides some much needed vitamins in your body and it can help with your chronic pain. It provides the lift in spirit to go along with that breath of fresh air.

Vitamin C

My mom has always told me to drink my orange juice. I have never liked orange juice because it leaves an acidic taste in my throat and a sick-to-my-stomach feeling. So I take Vitamin C instead. It can help reduce swelling as well as build your immune system, and we can use all the help we can get where Fibro is concerned.

Sam-E

This one I found on the internet.

I was looking for something that could help the Fibro joint pain and Sam-E kept coming up. I researched it thoroughly and found that many people take it for depression in lieu of a prescribed medication.

You should always talk to your doctor about replacing prescriptions with a natural supplement as natural supplements can have just as many side effects as a prescription. But if you have a doctor who is supportive of Fibromyalgia he will be interested in anything that may work for you and will have hopefully done his own research.

Upon looking into Sam-E further I saw that not only does it help with the moods caused by Fibro; it can actually help with the joint pain.

Many people take 1600 mg. of Sam-E which can be very expensive. A couple of medical notes I came across regarding Sam-E report that it builds in your system. What you may have needed in the beginning isn't what you might need in the long run.

In short, Sam-E is S-adenosylmethionine which is a naturally occurring molecule that is produced by your body. People who have an imbalance of healthy emotions can sometimes have very low levels of Sam-E in their system. Take Sam-E and you will be replenished with this much needed molecule should you be lacking it.

Sam-E has not been expensive for me. As I mentioned earlier, I am highly sensitive to typical dosage amounts. I bought a package of

Sam-E and took my pill cutter, reducing one 400 mg tablet into eight 50 mg sections. These were enteric coated so I wrapped each section in a piece of saran wrap to keep the moisture out.

An enteric coated pill keeps the insides of the pill protected from moisture so it doesn't lose its potency, but I have found that if I wrap them up they stay intact.

The directions say to take Sam-E on an empty stomach which gets it into your system without being diluted with food. But having a sensitive digestive system I took my first 50 mg tablet with my food once a day. After four days I increased the dose to 100 mg. I didn't have the normal gastrointestinal discomfort that can be associated with Sam-E by taking it with my food.

I worked my way up to 100 mg twice a day with food. This has helped me for the better. Joint pain is minimal and I feel more like my old self. I wouldn't do without it now.

They don't yet know the long term effects of Sam-E on the body. One day a week I skip my Sam-E so I can give my body a rest, and then I start again the next day. When you buy the Sam-E in 400 mg tablet packs and then divide each 400 mg tablet for use over a two day period, your Sam-E package will last you for over two months. That comes to less than twenty dollars a month.

Of course, not everyone could get by on the lower dose. But do remember that the Sam-E does build in the system. Many people encounter stomach irritations in the second week of taking Sam-E because of this buildup. That's why it's important to start out with a lesser dose. And yes, I still take it with food. I'm not up to hanging out in the bathroom with my crossword puzzles.

Sam-E works fine for me on a full stomach. I take it in the morning and the afternoon, but not at night as it has the propensity to keep you up at night.

Some say they get the anxiety jitters when they begin taking it, but I started with a low dose just to make sure it didn't happen to me.

You know, there's nothing quite like waking up in the morning and feeling like Snow White—without a care in the world and the birds singing. That's what Sam-E has done for me. It brings me back into the balance of who I am.

The real 'me' is inside this body, and I catch glimpses of her on my good days. And the good days now outweigh those bad Fibro days a hundred to one.

Omega 3 Fish Oil

I take fish oil because it helps minimize the nerve sensitivity as well as helping with my judgment, reasoning, my memory, and perceptions. This alone is a reason to take Fish Oil. You can now recognize family and friends! No more saying, "Hey You!" to your own kids. The kids will appreciate this, and so will you.

B-12

The vitamin B-12 has brought up my energy level and also helps with the tingling sensations and the tenderness throughout the body. It also boosts the Sam-E in your system.

This might be why I am able to get by with just the minimal amount of Sam-E. That's speculation, of course, but again, I just observe and do what works for me. I use the time released B-12 so that it is continually going through my system. I take it in the morning so it doesn't interrupt my sleep patterns.

There's a point where you feel as if all you do is think about the pills that you have to take, but it becomes a part of your morning routine just like brushing your teeth. So don't curse your supplements and pills. Do what you've got to do and then go about your day. Life is about living.

Do whatever you do to keep the body

going while you take care of the other parts of you that are just as important; like your mental state and feeling good in spite of Fibro.

When you are diagnosed with Fibro find out all you can about it and what has worked for others. Base your own symptoms on what they may have to say and keep doing research. But once you've got a handle on it, don't obsess over it.

Get educated on Fibromyalgia and once you begin to find a routine that works for you, begin living life. Don't put it off.

From time to time look at what's changed for you due to your Fibro research. But don't make it the end-all be-all for the rest of your life. Life is worth living.

You may have Fibro, but it's just a part of your daily life; it isn't what you're supposed to continually focus on. Understand Fibro and the limits for the day, but know that they could change tomorrow. There's always tomorrow or—in the case of Fibro—the next minute.

Korean Ginseng

Oh, that lovely Fibro fog. You wake up feeling as if you're in a tunnel. You know that your brain is in there somewhere, but you're sure that it's gone on vacation. You can't think clearly or even remember what your husband just said.

You tell yourself to focus and then you listen, but you can only hear through the tunnel. Any kind of jumping light puts you deeper into the tunnel, and before you know it you get so agitated that you want to head off to a corner and close your eyes thinking maybe you're having some kind of enlightening moment but all you get is...."DUH!"

I would say that this is one of the most frustrating Fibro symptoms.

I have always been a Type-A personality, getting it all done and then some, working from the wee hours in the morning to the late hours of the night—all the time enjoying and pushing myself.

I've co-written book after book on positive thought that took much longer than they should have simply because of the Fibro fog. It's as if the brain just went to mush. Sometimes the fog lifts after a few hours, and sometimes it decides to hang around for days. No matter what, it decides what I will or will not be doing for the day.

I have now created two lists for myself when working: One is for Fibro Fog Day, and the other is for the real Beth McCain brain day.

I refuse to give it any more attention than that and instead of waking up and wondering I wake up with a plan. It may be a sluggish plan, but it's a plan.

Korean Ginseng has helped me with my Fibro fog. My memory is much clearer and I remember faces more easily. The Korean Ginseng helps with my detail oriented work and my energy. Once I started taking it I began to have less Fibro Fog Days and more of the Real Beth McCain Days.

I guess what I'm trying to say is research; find out what might work for you, and then give it a try. If it works then let others know so that they can try it as well. We have to stick together and find something that will relieve the symptoms of Fibromyalgia.

And please remember, when even thinking about taking any of these supplements or prescriptions, to research the side effects. We are all different and one pill that might help one person and may not help another. Many people experience other conditions to be cautions of as well. Always check with your doctor before trying any of this for yourself.

Effexor

My family has background in FM and it seems that some of my own ancestors had this crazy condition. Many suffered and moved to the ocean air hoping that would help their physical body.

We are fortunate in this world today that we have some answers and I'm sure down the road there will be many answers for Fibromyalgia but until then it is 'trial and error' with our lifestyle and well as what we take to help the symptoms.

I had become agitated and the chronic pain and soreness put FM in my foreground instead of the background. Then my doctor put me on Effexor. At first I couldn't believe it. I'm on an anti depressant? What? I'm not depressed (even though many FM patients can be) but I wasn't myself that was for sure.

She told me that Effexor has been found to help FM patients. But not just for depression, but for pain. They have found that the prescription Effexor helps to suppress the nerves that are troubling the FM patient and therefore helping with some of the symptoms. My doctor said she wished they hadn't called most of the anti depressant 'anti depressants' because they have found that many of the so called anti depressants can help a myriad of problems in the human body. As FM patients some of us do not have enough serotonin in the brain and Effexor fits the bill.

When I started Effexor I became shaky and started sweating profusely. I called the doctor and she said, "Okay... You have to stick it out. It always is a little worse at first. Let's get you to open the capsule and sprinkle half on your food in the morning. As your body gets used to it we will increase it to the full dose." Oh and by the way—again—I am on the lowest dose that is available. Between the Sam-E and Effexor I have found some wonderful things that have happened.

Once my body got used to Effexor I began to notice a difference in about three weeks. The fog began to lift from my brain. I was able to get past the brain fog. My pain decreased some and the agitation began to leave.

So why not take a higher dose of either Sam-E or Effexor? Because like I have said, a million times over I want to eventually get beyond all of the pills and would prefer to just have over the counter.

If I just went with Sam-E the expense would be astronomical and if I just went with Effexor I don't like all the research I have seen on trying to wean off of it. By taking the low doses I know that I can from time to time see if I can get off of things if my body is in a better place with FM. (I always let my doctor know if I do this) They will tell me if they think it is not a good time so always keep in communication with your doctor and natural practitioners.

There is nothing better than having that brain fog lifted some. That is one of my biggest symptoms that I would love to get rid of and Effexor as well as Sam-E make me feel much clearer and less pain.

Ibuprofen

I don't take Ibuprofen on a daily basis; only as needed. Sometimes the pain feels like an inflammation instead of the usually elusive shooting or burning pains and it will occasionally work.

I want to stress that even though it sounds as if I am taking a mound of pills, I'm the type who prefers not to. I want my body to work on its own, but there's a point where the pain of Fibro takes front stage instead of lying dormant in the background. And when it affects my daily life I will try anything I believe may work. Some doctors say the Ibuprofen doesn't do anything for Fibro, but I'll say that when I have one of those Fibro headaches it definitely does the trick.

Sinus medication with Guaifenesin

I often wake up with a stuffy nose. This has happened all my life and I've been tested for allergies. I do have a few of the more common allergies, but the sinus headaches used to keep me from being able to work when I was younger.

I started taking sinus congestion medication and it seemed to get rid of the stuffiness. I now realize it has Guaifenesin in it and research shows that Guaifenesin is being used to treat Fibromyalgia, usually in larger doses by prescription. But the severe sinus congestion and pain medications contain acetaminophen, phenylephrine, and Guaifenesin and are sold over the counter.

The amount of Guaifenesin is 200 mg per caplet and I take two each morning. This takes care of the sinuses well enough, but it also has a great side attribute that helps with the general aching of the body caused by Fibro.

Some medical professionals say the relief is tendered because of the acetaminophen, but I have tried the congestion caplet without Guaifenesin and it does nothing for me. Maybe this is something that can help for you.

Anything that will clear up the head is all right with me.

The Guaifenesin therapy is currently under scrutiny with reports saying that it doesn't help Fibro. It's also been stated that the minute amount I take couldn't help a flea, but I'm just telling you what works for me. My particular sensitivity to doses of medication may be a plus factor in my case.

The Guaifenesin dose isn't huge which is better for our bodies so as not to be dependent on a pill. If we have to take medication (for right now anyway), the smaller the dose the better, as far as I'm concerned. But be aware that if the smaller dose doesn't work you should talk to your doctor about a taking regular dose.

We're all different so I'm always interested in what doctors say will absolutely not work when they don't even know what Fibromyalgia actually is. There are speculations, yes, but until I hear a bonafide, straight-out, one hundred percent 'this is what Fibromyalgia is' answer, I'm going to continuing to seek what can work for me.

Omeprazole
Yet another doctor and more tests.

I had had upper and lower GI problems for most of my life which were diagnosed as IBS and acid reflux disease. So when I went in for my forty-something GI tests it amazed me to learn that I didn't have acid reflux or anything else. Yet I still had GI spasms as well as extreme heartburn.

When the day came when I finally was diagnosed with Fibromyalgia it all made sense. All these symptoms mimicked something else.

Maybe the medicine that is used for some of the mimicked diseases and conditions might work on a Fibro patient. I was given Omeprazole which is Prevacid and it worked like a charm for another one of my symptoms.

Wow, another symptom taken care of! Five hundred more to go! Or at least that's what it felt like. But I was beginning to feel better as I ticked off each symptom, replacing it with some kind of supplement.

Hyland's Nerve Tonic

Okay, I know this sounds like something your grandma would have bought off the back of a peddler's wagon. But I would have chased the wagon down if I'd known how well it works.

Hyland's is a homeopathy company that provides a range of remedies. The long and short of how homeopathy works is that a small very minute trace of what ails you (or what might be an antidote to what you have) is formulated into a teeny-tiny round pellet. They look and taste like sugar but they work very well.

There are many doctors that don't believe in homeopathy but it has worked for my family for many years. When my kids were little they always responded to homeopathy for ear aches and the usual childhood ailments.

Hyland produces a product called Nerve Tonic. It's supposed to help the body be able to relieve stress and tension naturally. These are actual caplets and not pellets and they help relieve the agitation that accompanies Fibro.

When you are in chronic pain you can become agitated and the agitation can create even more symptoms. By reducing or getting rid of the agitation, your senses calm down as do the aches in your body. I am all for encouraging the agitation to take a hike.

Valerian Root

Here is an herb that has helped improve my sleep cycle. It calms and relaxes me and I take it right before I go to bed. I take this one religiously. I take Baclofen on the days when the muscle spasms just won't behave but Valerian

Root is the one I use the most for improving sleep. I notice a difference if I don't take it and I find that I toss and turn much more than usual without it.

Again, not every Fibro patient experiences the sensitivity to these kinds of supplement and medications, but most do. Don't write off a medication that's been prescribed to you just because the usual dose that most people take puts you to sleep or makes you sweat even worse.

Ask your doctor if you can start at a much lower dose and see if it works for you. We want to get back to feeling good but you also don't want to rule out any kind of medication that may help. So another week of feeling bad won't matter if you slowly work the medication up to the dosage that works for you.

When talking to your doctor about sensitivity to medication make sure, if they do prescribe medication to you, that it can be easily cut into halves or fourths with a pill cutter. Some of them may come as a capsule (which I just open up, use half, and save the rest for the next day). Again, everything works differently for different people. You and the doctor just have to discover the right formula for you through medication, supplements, and lifestyle changes that will help you cope and put Fibro in the background of your life.

CHAPTER THREE

Getting Through Today!

My hearing was so astute that I could hear every noise within two hundred yards. I would stop and listen. "Did you hear that?" I would ask my husband. "I don't hear a thing."

"It sounds like maybe...Lassie is trying to tell me something. Timmy fell down the well?"

He would roll his eyes. Every noise from the spatula scraping the frying pan to the cat licking his fur sent my nerves and muscles into spasms.

I could never understand why I couldn't listen to music like the rest of them. When I would hear music it would be as if my system went into overload. Music always had to be quiet and ethereal. I couldn't listen to anything over a whisper, yet everyone else couldn't hear a thing. I needed the television so low that no one else wanted to watch television with me or they would strain to hear even one word. After researching FM I found others who understood where I was coming from. In some ways finding out that I had FM gave me a feeling of freedom that all these things I had experienced through my lifetime were part of an illness and not me just being the sensitive type. I now knew why!

I could barely step into a room full of light and you could forget about being out in the sun. The sun dappling through the trees sent my eyes into a frenzy, trying to get away from the burning light. I was able to smell any and everything but on a potent level.

"Do you smell that?" I would ask my daughter.

"What are you talking about, Mom?"

"The gas smell coming from the house five doors down?" Again I got the rolling of the eyes.

What was I going to do with these kinds of super powers? What could I do with a keen sense of smell? I could tell if someone used the bathroom five hours ago. Now *that's* a skill to have. What about hearing the grass grow? I had to think this through. But not only that, the slightest touch sent me into muscle-like spasms, as if kryptonite had been placed on my skin. So, human contact was the nemesis. No, this isn't superpowers, this is kryptonite. My body didn't feel like my own. There was some unknown force that was causing my body to repel even itself.

So how do I handle the days where all my senses are heightened? This is the one symptom that doesn't seem to leave my side. I can hear so clearly with such crashing force that I'm surprised I'm not being used for some secret spy mission to listen through walls. The 'bright light' feelings come and go and my sense of being touched is continually heightened.

I have found that if I put cotton in my ears it buffers the loud sounds I hear and it even helps 'sinus plugged' ears and burning neck pain. The cotton isn't annoying like ear plugs and actually feels quite nice. It has saved me many times while in public. The sounds can become overwhelming. When my family asks what it is like to have bat sonar I tell them imagine turning up the volume to ten on your CD player and then add in a hundred times more. That about covers it.

I use good old sunglasses when it comes to the light and have transitional lenses for that very purpose. I got the darkest black I could and it has helped me tolerate going in the sun or being under bright lights.

Now what have I done for the sense of touch? This is a tricky one. You want your family to hug you and you want to be able to hug them back but sometimes just the slightest touch—no matter how much love it comes from—just plain hurts. We have what we call the Fibro pat if I'm having a particularly touch sensitive day. The Fibro pat is a light baby hug with the words 'I love you' attached to it.

It's hard to understand if you haven't experienced it but the slightest touch is like someone punching you with full force. It doesn't leave a mark but it sends shooting aches and pains throughout the whole body. Family and friends have to be told what is different about you these days.

I remember a particular doctor I went to whose nurse had what I thought was personality clash with me. She complained and looked disheveled as if she didn't care about her patients or her job. She seemed continually agitated every time we saw her. After being diagnosed with Fibro I called the doctor for something. This nurse answered and I struck up a conversation with her about my diagnosis and she told me, "I have Fibromyalgia as well. It can be difficult, can't it?"

I assumed I knew this woman and thought I had a personality clash when in fact she actually had Fibro. I realized that she must have been having one of the harder days. Not that you want to go around announcing to the world, "Hey, I have Fibromyalgia! Stay clear!" But be aware of others around you who may not be able to understand what you are going through, just as we may not be able to understand what they are going through in life. Let's give each other the benefit of the doubt and the unconditional love and support that goes with it. That will get all of us through.

Our systems seem to be sensitive to every outer sensitivity. Something that has helped me is to make lists of what is important for the day. I use to be a multi-tasker but have found that picking one or two things on my list and finishing them keeps me from feeling overwhelmed. That overwhelming feeling is a precursor to a Fibro flare.

Take one task at a time and then take a break moving on with ease and not out of stress. Try not to be over stimulated. When you are in a room and it is buzzing with excitement and people are talking, glasses are clinking, and music is blaring, step out for a moment to clear the mind. All of that overstimulation is like murder on an FM person but stepping out for a moment helps your nervous system to center once again.

If you are in a meeting or in a position where you can't just leave, think of the calm that resides within you and go there before you speak or get your system into over stimulation. Focus on one thing at a time, all the while maintaining a center. Remember, we are learning to listen to our bodies first and the stress and the outside world second.

So in times of stress take a short break and focus elsewhere. You can always come back to the stress but step aside for some time. When things get too much to handle remember it is all in your reaction of how you respond. Change your response or find the calm within yourself and do your best to shorten the type of stress you might be encountering. Less stress is best. If you're heading into a stressful situation do your best to relax and think it through in the calm of your mind first.

YIPPEE! A Crisis!

A crisis would appear and I'd become superwoman; able to leap off buildings in a single bound taking care of everyone and everything around me—and then I slowed down.

After a particularly grueling stressed filled day I would go home and crash. And the crash is what would bring on the symptoms. I looked forward to getting someone out of a mess just for the adrenaline rush so that I could get beyond the ever present soreness and pain.

One day I was feeling flu-ish I decided to take a walk with my girls. Sometimes the mild exercise helps the joint pain. It so happened that as we walked the horse next door was excited to see us. It had to do with the apple my daughter was holding.

I was walking with my shoulders slumped, too tired and painful to lift them up until…the horse tried to jump the fence. It knocked my then nine-year-old to the ground and part of the fence fell on her. Immediately my adrenaline kicked in and I stepped in front of the horse to keep him from trampling my baby. I became Supermom as I stuck my chest out and growled 'back off' in the horse's ear all the while protecting my daughter. The horse's front hoofs landed on my chest but I didn't feel a thing. I felt as if I pushed that two ton horse back with my whole body. It was the adrenaline push racing through my body.

Once it backed off I picked up my daughter who had a gash in her shoulder from the barbed wire fence. My shoulders were back, I had more energy than an army of men, and I was able to get her home unharmed. We replayed the scenario in our minds and began to laugh. Did that really happen?

I looked down and there were two horse hoof prints on my shirt for proof. The next morning I was flat on my back once again from the symptoms. Crisis took away the symptoms but they always came back in full force. Supermom became SuperFibroMom once again. The adrenaline rush strikes again, but remember after that adrenaline comes the letdown. I have found the best antidote is to find the calm within.

The more I focus on my breathing and keep my peace within myself I don't get the huge adrenaline rush that sends me into a *Throwdown with Fibro* week. Part of lessening the symptoms is to learn how to take care of your own self first. I have always been the one everyone goes to for answers.

"What should I do today? Let's go ask Beth!"

"Can you take care of my four-hour problem before you go eat, Beth?"

"You're going for a walk. Can I go along so I can tell you all about it?"

"YES, YES, YES! I want to take care of all your problems! I have solutions just for you! Yes, I will sacrifice anything to help you out!" Yet my body is yelling, very loudly, "NO. You have to take care of you first!" So what did I used to do? Ignore myself. I became a driven passionate martyr. *"I can do it. Even if I feel like crap I will help you move your whole house all by myself."* Out of the side of my mouth, *"Quiet, body. I am helping. I don't have time for you."* It would whimper. I guess it got tired of whimpering and took on a voice.

"You are not going to ignore me any longer!"

What am I saying here? There is nothing wrong with asking for help when you need it and there is nothing wrong with saying no. Find the balance so that your body can feel the balance. If you need a jar opened because today your hands just can't do it, don't go ahead and destroy your hands so that you don't have to ask someone else for help. Make sure to keep a good balance and not go from martyr to witch.

"I NEED HELP HERE! Can't you see I'm HURTING?!"

People will be running and hiding from that particular Fibro witch. If you are having a particularly hard day make sure you let your loved ones know. Do what you can on your own (without pushing) and ask for help when you need it. Taking care of your body (and *you*) is the top priority when you aren't feeling well when it comes to Fibromyalgia.

If someone doesn't understand that, don't let it get you down. Maybe Fibro was put in my life to teach me to be good to myself and not ignore my body. I used to be the go getter and wouldn't stop until it was all done and then start again the next morning. Being everywhere at once is highly overrated. My life now has more balance and Fibro made me see that. Fibro took me in a direction that I had never gone; and that was within 'me'.

What doesn't it do?

I was and still do pore over books constantly and search the internet for answers. I fully expect one day to Google 'fibromyalgia' and see a wonder pill that takes care of it all. But until then we do our best to figure it all out.

One source describes Fibromyalgia as:

> **A chronic disorder characterized by widespread musculoskeletal pain, fatigue, and multiple tender points that occurs in precise, localized areas, particularly in the neck, spine, shoulders, and hips; also may cause sleep disturbances, morning stiffness, irritable bowel syndrome, anxiety, and other symptoms.**

And the doctors wonder why we come in asking for help.

Fibromyalgia is getting much more attention than it used to. It started out being ignored but more and more people, mostly women, began to come in with symptoms. It was deemed a disorder that was stress induced and worthy of the classic hypochondriac.

Do you have any idea what it is like to go into a doctor's office with very real symptoms only to be told that maybe you're just under a little stress? It makes you feel ignored, alone, and crazy until you realize that it isn't you, it is the doctor who is crazy, ignored, and alone. Why them? Because they are crazy to think anyone would make up these kinds of symptoms, they are ignored because you are no longer going to listen to that particular doctor, and they are alone because you're changing to a doctor who will listen and help. **No one has to put up with not being heard.** "Hey doc! No one puts Baby in a corner!"

Find someone who will listen. You will have to take the initiative and be your own champion but when you find the right doctor who gives you the FM diagnosis, you will feel relief, well, until you realize that now you're going to have to listen to your body. No more ignoring what it is telling you.

Just finding a doctor who encourages and supports your journey with Fibro is a huge boost. You want answers and you deserve answers. Keep looking for someone who will listen and guide you.

How about clown shoes?

For years I was convinced that I was wearing the wrong kind of shoes. No matter what I wore my feet always hurt, ached, and burned by the end of the day and then they started burning and aching in the morning after I had a nice sleep.

I searched for and found shoes that wouldn't hug my feet so tightly but I found that if I really wanted shoes that felt good, I should invest in a good pair of clown shoes. They stay on the heel but are big and bulky around the front without touching your toes. A perfect Fibro shoe! But alas, I would then have to join the circus and that is a whole other story.

There are two things I do for the burning, aching feet.

I change shoes often and I take my shoes *off* just as often. A shoe that is like a sandal or clog (without a back) didn't work for me. If my feet have to do any hanging on to a sandal or a clog they begin to burn and hurt from the work it takes from the toes.

My toes can't hang on to the shoe properly because they can't take any kind of repetitive movement so I buy Uggs or some kind of boot that is nice and soft on the inside in a slightly bigger size than my feet. I also love a great pair of running shoes as long as they are light and not too heavy and feel 'just right.' If a shoe is too heavy it again sets my feet on fire.

A running shoe is made to support your feet when running but they also provide great arch support that is needed when dealing with the heat of the feet. When I go out I bring an extra pair of shoes with me and if my feet start giving me trouble just the change of the shoes lessens the burning and aching. What works best is taking off my shoes if I am in a sitting position. If I'm in the car you will find my shoeless feet up on the dashboard and if you find me in a restaurant and look under the table, you will see my shoeless feet. Just that short amount of time can give me hours of relief.

I can't stand on my feet long but I also can't sit for too long so I am in constant motion to keep the aching at bay but a girl's got to do what a girl's got to do!

I'll wake up in the morning feeling as if I can't move. I ache all over and reach over for my sinus meds. My nose is stuffed and my head is congested. I've changed detergents. I've got an air purifier. I've slept with Vick's Vapo-Rub under my nose. I've got all the normal things you would use to get rid of all the above. Some mornings are good but most mornings it takes a lot to get me up and once I'm up and move my stiff body into the bathroom it begins to subside a little.

Then comes the 'which bra is it today' dilemma. You see, with Fibro any constricting clothing makes your day, well, constricted. Your body starts the uncomfortable burning feeling and then goes into the "uncomfortable, have to get this off" feeling.

I remember in high school when we were all trading clothes a friend of mine was a size five. I wanted to be in that size five but, alas, I was a seven. I suffered through the high heels not realizing that everyone wasn't having the aching problems I was and I ignored my body, doing whatever I wanted. Hey, that's what being a goofy teen is all about!

But one day I had it in my mind that I was going to fit into those size five jeans. I laid on the bed on my back pulling and pulling those yellow ditto jeans on. I got them over my hips and with a lot of sucking in was able to snap and zip them. Now to get up.

I rolled over on my side and stood. I applauded myself. I fit in a size five jeans! Then the first uncomfortable spasms arose. My arms tightened and I couldn't unsnap the pants. My hands froze. I then took my thumbs and whittled the snap apart and peeled the jeans off. That incident left me in pain for days. A measly little pants pull!

I figured everybody felt like that after trying on a pair of pants that were too small, and I left it at that. I didn't want anything to mess up my fun-filled life as a teen. But I'll never forget thinking, "No matter what size I am, I am happy with because I don't ever want to wear something that made me feel like that ever again."

So here I am staring at my three 'over the shoulder boulder holder' drawers. One drawer is filled with bras that are sports bra-like that are as comfortable as can be, as little constraint as possible. They may not make my girls look the best but they make me feel better and I have found that is all that matters.

My husband asked on a particular light bra day, "Why not just go without one?" He found out yet one more ache and what it led to.

"If I go without one the heaviness of my boobs pull on my neck and back and then…"

"No further explanation needed," he said. "I got it."

Next is drawer number two. That is what I opted for today. This drawer is full of the supportive cushioned strapped bras. They have enough give to be comfortable and they support well. This drawer is for the days where I can handle some constrictions on the body. We'll call them my perky boob bras.

The next drawer I only look into. There is one bra that is a size smaller than what I am, that is all lacy without much support, but is pretty. I pet this one from time to time knowing that it is there. Maybe one day.

I have drawers for all of my different kinds of pants as well. I buy jeans with spandex so that they have a little give. Yes, it's nice that they have give for that extra piece of chocolate cake I may have had, but they also make it so that on some days you can wear pants with a snap and a zipper, and with that extra give they aren't quite so constrictive.

And then there are pants that just have elastic at the waist. I never thought I would be wearing 'those' kind of pants. You know, the ones you see sweet little old ladies wearing along with their light-up sweatshirts, but I'm telling you, I now know why they wear them.

They are comfortable and some days comfortable is what you have to do when it comes to Fibro. I usually wear a long turtleneck or sweater over the top so you can't see my granny pants. Don't be embarrassed if you have to buy sizes bigger than you really are. No one will be looking at the tag and you will have one less constriction torturing your body. Cut out the tags if the size bothers you. I cut out the tags anyways because my body can't handle the scratch of a tag.

Do I have a "pants on the pedestal" pair of pants like my lacy bra? I sure do! They're just waiting for me... I can see it now...

When you have Fibromyalgia every little detail matters, from the pants to the bras, from the shoes to your glasses. It has to be non constrictive to make your body feel less tight. And you will get to wear those designer jeans. It just depends on the day.

Do my hands look fat?

We're going out for a full day of shopping and movie watching. So I get my Fibro pack ready: soft gushy Uggs, layering of clothes for the hot and cold moments, a scarf for the sub-zero neck cold, socks that don't cut into my skin, muscle spasm meds, glasses that change from light to dark on their own, book for if I have to stay in the car from pain, earphones and music for if I have to stay in the car and the outer noise is too loud for me to be able to read. That just about covers it.

I get into the car with all my regalia and within minutes my outer sweater comes off. The defrost button is on high heat so that we can see out of the car, so my Fibro body is having a hard time adjusting.

Next is the scarf. I take off my shoes to get my feet comfortable before any Fibro business begins, and I drink nice cool water to relax the body. Five seconds later the car is all defrosted and then the process goes backwards. The shoes go back on, the scarf wraps back around the neck, and the sweater is buttoned tight all the while there's an underlying fatigue, soreness, and aching all over the body. I now am drinking my half cup of coffee to ward off the cold or else it will start up the spasms.

I avert my eyes from the dabbling light that seems to set off spasms. The Baclofen has helped immensely with the spasms throughout my whole body and I keep monitoring myself throughout the day.

I love going out. I really do, and Fibro can mess with your whole day... if you let it. We enjoy our ride into town and I put on, take off, put on, take off knowing that if I don't listen to the body it will begin to manifest in a different painful way. I'm used to it.

I sit and thank the Universe that I have a sweater and scarf to take on and off. Even one that I like. I laugh and enjoy myself in the car with my family or friends and do what my body says to do. No complaining, no yelling at how stupid it all seems; just acceptance and another part of the routine. Then we get to the store. This is when it really gets fun!

I put on my sweater and find the nearest cart. I drop my purse (that seems as if it weighs two tons) into the cart. It's actually very light, but tell my shoulder and body that. It feels nice to lean on the cart and I look forward to going in and interacting. Enjoying time to do what girls do.

The walk from the car to the store seems okay today and I walk in the doors. The heat hits and the fluorescent lights begin to do their work. The sunglasses are no longer dark, but clear like my regular prescription glasses. I'm feeling pretty good and start to work my way through the box store.

The lights begin to make me feel even dizzier than what I normally feel. The spasms begin and my hands and feet begin to tingle and shake. Then comes the Fibro Fog. What was it I was supposed to buy? I know myself well. I pull out my list and begin to get through the store. I have even written down which debit card to use. No one knows what I am going through. I pass other people and stop and chat.

I smile at babies passing by and do my best to enjoy being in the store. I help a little elderly man find his fiber and I go to pick up the cat food. With each step I take I realize I probably should have stayed in the car, but then the adventurous person who sits inside me says, "We are not going to let Fibromyalgia turn us into a recluse, are we?"

My wedding rings tighten on my hand and my feet begin to feel like I'm walking flat footed. The fatigue hits and I can barely get to the cashier before getting into the car and wondering where I picked up these puffed up Mickey Mouse hands.

I pull off my boots and my sweater and rest my head on the back of the seat. My glasses have turned dark and I wait for the pain and aching to subside. It doesn't. It becomes part of my day. The exhaustion is overwhelming. You can't make it go away.

We go to have lunch and my friends are looking at me with concern. This isn't Beth. She is the go-getting laugh-a-minute gal. I straighten my back and do my best to enjoy who is around me. I keep focusing on what is good around me instead of the mean little monster poking at me from within. I keep shifting my focus to what I like around me; how I can enjoy the moment and keep the monster at bay as best I can.

I shuffle through the rest of the day and congratulate myself for doing my best. This isn't an everyday occurrence. I have days where I feel like Maria from the *Sound of Music*. Singing from the hilltops and dancing *Do Re Mi* but I even watch my *Do Re Mi* because if I don't it becomes Do Re *Don't* and Fibro lets me know it pretty quick. I guess what I'm saying is that it doesn't go completely away.

It is always in the background but I'm good with that. It's when it jumps to center stage that it affects my whole day. I have found my best defense is to listen to my body's signals. If I'm feeling just the least bit tired I step down and sit in a relaxed position.

If I can't go to every store and lunch too, I don't mind sitting one out. If I'm in the mood to whip up a cheese soufflé but Fibro is letting itself known, I save the soufflé for a better time. And there is a better time. Once you get the hang of listening to your body and respect Fibromyalgia for what it is, then you begin to see a light at the end of the tunnel. No more commanding the body to do what you say.

Now it's time to take the backseat and listen because when you do, you will find that

Fibro can be manageable. I am fortunate that I am able to work from my home and pick my own hours. For those of you working a nine-to-five job (either on your feet or behind a desk) you will have to find your own method of coping.

Make sure to not stand in one place for too long or sit behind your desk for hours at a time. It's important to move the body in a different position with Fibro. Sit for twenty minutes then walk around for a few. Just changing that position from a repetitive movement seems to loosen up my Fibro body.

Tender points!
(More like Round Ten in the boxing ring)

"So does this hurt?" the doctor asked.

"Here let me get my nails out of the ceiling," I screeched.

I had no idea that there were tender points until I stepped into the neurologist's office. When she touched the back of my neck it felt like someone had put a knife through my back. I had always known that I had a sensitive neck and that no one—yes no one—was privy to the neck.

When my husband and I got married he accepted the fact that I was just not one of those people who like my neck rubbed but he didn't really know the true reason. My neck was always tense and on fire and if you messed with anything around my neck you would suffer the consequences. I felt that although I was a bit of a 'Type A' personality I was good at releasing stress through exercise and meditation. Throughout my life I thought maybe it was tension or that I might have pulled something but there was a point where I realized that I could not have pulled my back and neck every single day of my life.

Another moment sticks out that I remember where I should have recognized Fibromyalgia. They say that Fibro can come on after a traumatic experience such as an accident or any kind of physical/mental trauma.

When I was pregnant with my second child I expected the birth to be easy. My first labor and birth had been a breeze and I didn't expect anything less with my second child. I was told over and over again that I looked like I was pregnant with twins. It felt like it. I couldn't see my feet but the pregnancy had been just a dream.

I craved steak and potatoes with this one and truly enjoyed my pregnancy. I was overdue by three weeks and was feeling a bit like a beach ball when I woke one morning with contractions. I thought, "Well, tonight at this time I'll have myself a little sweetheart."

I continued with the contractions all through the day and way into the night. The contractions got to be about five minutes apart and we decided to head to the hospital. We checked in and the doctor checked me.

"You're almost fully dilated," the doctor said. "Just keep walking the hospital floor and you'll be having a baby within the hour."

I breathed and walked and walked and breathed and seven hours later was still walking and breathing. But now the baby was wanting out. I wasn't quite fully dilated.

I went into transitional labor where the contractions are one on top of the other. This went on for hours. I was worn out and had exceeded my first son's labor time by forty-eight hours. When it was time to push it took forever for the baby's head to come down.

I heard the doctor say the word 'huge baby' and saw the scissors. Snip, snip, tear. I didn't feel a thing but I had run out of steam and my body's adrenaline was running thin. The baby came in at nine pounds fourteen ounces. My body didn't know what to do.

My newborn son was swollen and I was exhausted but I had done it. Come to find out I shouldn't have. He should have been taken Cesarean.

My body shook and began coming down off the adrenaline high. You may say, "Well of course she was exhausted. That's normal." But what happened after wasn't normal and I can say that it was probably my first full bonafide Fibro attack.

When I stood up for the first time after birth my legs, arms, and neck ached. Every bone in my body felt as if it had been hit by a truck. I figured after all the heavy duty pushing it was just a normal feeling, even though I had never experienced it with my first childbirth and labor.

I walked to the bathroom and the dizziness hit. The nurse caught me as I passed out. When I awoke I had never felt this bad in my life. They sent me home with instructions and my son, and I didn't know how I was going to do any of it. The pain and fatigue through my body only got worse as the weeks went by.

Many words were thrown around: 'Post Depression', 'Baby Exhaustion' — but this was different. This went on for six months after he was born. The trauma of the birth had sent me into the first full-blown Fibro attack but I didn't find out until years later (twenty-five to be exact) what had really happened.

There is research that shows that Fibromyalgia is hereditary. I believe that in my family's case it's true. My mom remembers her mother telling her that there was nothing on her body that didn't hurt whenever someone touched her.

She complained of extreme fatigue as well, but back in those days they would say she had the vapors or that everyone was feeling that way with all the physical work that they had to do. I really wonder how many ancestors had this disorder and were given the brush off. We're fortunate that we now have people that are recognizing and treating this condition.

Maybe this has you thinking back to when this started for you, or maybe you remember the second it began for you. It doesn't matter when or where as much as it matters that you find relief and some treatment or at least some helpful tips on how to maintain a semblance of a life.

So where are the tender points, and what can you do so you don't feel like you're in round ten in the boxing ring? Don't let anyone touch them! Hee hee…

Let's begin where the tender points actually are.

There are eighteen tender points that you may not even be aware of. You may have widespread pain but had no idea that there are points on your body that are so tender that if someone just presses slightly, it will send you straight up to the ceiling.

You may not be sore in all those points but if you have eleven out of eighteen of the tender points it is one of the key factors in being diagnosed with Fibromyalgia.

Tender points are located:

- Right below your hairline there is a left or a right side of the back of the neck.

- Where your neck and should come together there is a left or a right tender point.

- Right between your shoulder blades on the left or right side of your spine.

- Right below your waist the left or right side of your back.

- The right or left on either side of your bottom right below your hipbones.

- On the front of your neck, left or right side, above your collarbone.

- On the right or left side of your chest, right below your collarbone.
- On the inside of each of your arms where your elbow bends.

- On the inside of your kneecaps area where it is fleshy.

Keep in mind that if you have only ten of the eighteen tender points this doesn't mean that you *don't* have Fibromyalgia. You could be having one of those days when you are less sore and it is manifesting in that way. Best to go in when you're having a full blown Fibro flare-up to have your tender points checked. But don't wait for one. Go in anyway and get to the bottom of what is going on so that you can start some kind of treatment.

    Sometimes a heating pad helps but most of the time I have found that stretching can relieve the tightness and some of the pain. My tender points don't hurt unless someone touches them. They are constantly sore and achy, but <u>that</u> I can manage.

    Changing positions is one of the ways I deal with them. Laying on one side for too long creates the super stabbing pain up and down and this affects the tender points but if I lay on one side and get that agitated feeling started I switch sides and it subsides.

This is how I sleep at night. My mind wakes up just long enough to tell me to flip other and change position. Do this during the day as well. Some minimal movement and stretching is beneficial to your Fibro.

Do your best to stand up and stretch. Getting your body to stretch doesn't sound like much but it does me a world of good. I am usually sitting at a computer nine hours out of a waking day. I get up and stretch every twenty minutes and I take a break at least three times and walk around. This does my body a world of good and it helps the stiffness and aching associated with Fibro.

But you just went 5 minutes ago!

"What is up with my bladder?" was a common thought that used to run through my mind. I seemed to have to pee all the time. I was checked for urinary infections, kidney infections, wichie-wachie-woo infections (at least that's what it began to sound like).

"You must have an overactive bladder," I was told when all else failed. This is another sign of Fibromyalgia. I attribute it to the spasms. Usually the bladder goes crazy when I'm having the spasm symptoms. This has calmed down since I started taking the Baclofen and the homeopathy remedy 'Nerve Tonic.' (every time I write down Nerve Tonic I imagine a Gypsy wagon!)

But even with the medication I am in the bathroom a lot. Just another wonderful effect to look forward to on one of those Fibro days.

All of my life I have had upper and lower GI problems. It started when I was in sixth grade and I missed a total of three months of school, on and off, due to nausea and IBS. Then it seemed to subside in my teen years and after my children were born, it came on like gangbusters.

There was diarrhea, constipation, nausea, bloating, heartburn, and spasms. I couldn't make it to the bathroom, and driving my kids to school required a trip to the bathroom at home, at the school, and back home again. You would have thought I would have been a size two as much as I went.

I had test after test in my twenties to find out what exactly was happening. I was told I had Irritable Bowel Syndrome.

I was given a classic checklist of things to do; Fiber, Imodium AD, Xanax (if needed), and a pat on the shoulder (ouch!). I took the fiber, abused the Imodium AD, and threw the Xanax in the trash. I felt like pills seemed to be the only answer and I had a choice in that. I have done my best to stay clear of any prescriptions unless the side effects were minimal and it wasn't addictive. I prefer the discomfort over the thought of taking something that might tell me I won't be able to stop. I had three small children, PTA meetings, work, and house payments. I spent more time in the bathroom than with my own kids, with no real answers.

I used to daydream of inventing a porta-potty that you could use right in the car for those 'just in case' moments. I knew every bathroom from our home town to the nearest big city. I used every one of them. Too bad they didn't offer frequent potty miles, because I would have been upgraded to first class!

I have been able to beat this symptom with relaxation techniques, psyllium seed husk fiber, and heartburn medication. I rarely have an episode of gastric proportion these days. But if I do I have my trusty invention the porta-potty 2000 (which is available in the Hefty trash bag aisle at the grocery store). It is a little added assurance for the just-in-case moments, as it seems that Fibro is a just-in-case disorder.

You never know how you're going to wake up in the morning. You can be fine one minute and down the next. You can then be down and a few hours later be up and running. I carry a bag full of 'just in case' with me so I can go about my day knowing that I'm prepared for anything Fibro throws at me.

Doctor Jekyll and Mister Hyde.

It feels as if you are at the bottom of a well. The sound seems to amplify and you just can't seem to get anyone to hear you down in the deep, dark hole.

"Hello? Anybody out there?"

Then someone from somewhere throws you a flashlight and now you have a little light that begins to grow as you come out of the hole. You don't always come out. Sometimes you feel as if you've been there for days and other times there's just a flash of the dark hole. No matter what, the mental symptoms of Fibromyalgia are the most confusing and frightening aspect of Fibro.

For someone who has always taken life by the reins, Fibro can really feel as if it has set you back. It's as if you are watching your body and mind take over and you just don't feel like yourself. The mind takes on what they call Fibro Fog, a time when you are confused, forget things, are agitated, and just plain aren't yourself.

It's as if your brain is the attic and all that clutter has finally taken over. It is so cluttered that you can't make heads nor tails of anything. You know what you want and need but you can't seem to express it. Words end up coming out backwards and you just can't seem to think of the word; that one word that will tell it all.

If I have to say there is a symptom of Fibro that frustrates me and keeps me asking 'why me' the most, it would be all of the problems associated with the mind.

You start out feeling foggy and progress to wanting to cry. You can't express yourself any other way. You begin to feel like you are on a carousel and you can't get off. You'd think you were drunk by the way your balance is off. You walk to one side thinking you're walking straight. I call it my Hunchback of Notre Dame walk, all hunched over and limping to one side.

Your sense of direction is nonexistent. You can have driven over and over again to the same restaurant and all of a sudden you can't remember which way to go. Your reasoning and figuring things out goes from hard to virtually impossible depending on the level of that day's Fibro flare.

You begin to worry that someone might notice and if they do you, that won't be able to explain to them what is going on. You begin to not want to go out without a trusty friend at your side because you're concerned that you may end up wandering down the street. There is enough of you there to know that what you are thinking is ludicrous, but you feel helpless and all those feelings for a 'take control' kind of person makes you feel so much less of the person that you know you are. One minute you are full of vim and vigor and the next minute you can barely remember your name.

You go to write and you can't spell or the words come out backwards. You decide you want to be alone to possibly clear your head but you also want people around 'just in case' (there's that phrase again for this unpredictable disorder). You might forget and take a pill twice. You feel alone as if no one could possibly understand what is happening to you.

"I'm not sick, I'm not sick... I'm not... What was I saying?"

Then comes the motherlode of all of them... the depression. Why wouldn't we be depressed? Some alien has taken over our bodies and we didn't get to even have a say so in it. You can't fight it or it gets worse.

You realize your life has been turned upside down yet you are still walking, breathing, and living some semblance of life. Doctors scoff and tell you it's stress and your family just can't quite understand.

Don't forget that there is **you** within all of this. You are not alone. There are many of us out there who experience what you are experiencing. It helps knowing that fact. It helps to know that someone believes you and is trying to help you. If you haven't found the right doctor then keep trying until you do.

Depression is a chemical imbalance. That is nothing to be ashamed of. And it seems that Fibromyalgia is a hormonal and chemical imbalance, so no wonder you have a looming depression. If you are put on an antidepressant remember this can be temporary and you can regain some balance in your body.

Some antidepressants can actually help joint pain, hot cold flashes, and fatigue as well. I wish they hadn't called them antidepressants. There is some kind of stigma attached to being depressed that I just don't get. It is a condition just like high blood pressure that can be helped, and antidepressants aren't used just for depression. They can also be used for myriad Fibromyalgia symptoms.

With depression, some of the neurochemicals in the brain are called serotonin, dopamine, and norepinephrine.

If these chemicals are not balanced, then you can run into problems. That's all you need, another symptom. So if you end up taking an antidepressant for your Fibromyalgia it can be helpful in many ways. Fibromyalgia is not you. You are just someone who happens to have Fibromyalgia. You are still here. You still have much purpose.

You just have to change a few things and begin to take care of your body, but that's it. It is your life and Fibro isn't going to stop you from being who you want to be. It has lessons within it to teach us to tolerate others who don't understand, to accept ourselves for who we are, to not be so hard on ourselves, and to take care of one's self inside and out.

Fibro shows you all these things. Fibromyalgia has made me a more compassionate person. Fibromyalgia has taught me to put my needs first and then take care of others. I sit with Fibro on the couch and laugh at its ludicrous ways of getting my attention. Don't worry Fibro, I won't forget you. I really do know you're there.

So what has helped me with the Fibro Fog? Sam-E, Korean Ginseng, and Vitamin D have helped some of my symptoms. I have yet to find something for the dizziness but I can cut through the fog when I am taking Sam-E and Effexor. Details came back to me when taking Korean Ginseng, and my doctor recommended Vitamin D. I use the lightest makeup foundation you can find, (look for white as ghost foundation) and that is what I use which means I use a lot of sun block, which means my skin isn't getting much in the way of the sun which means without the sun you can get depressive.

Lack of Vitamin D can make you feel melancholy, especially living in a state where it rains most of the time. So that's why I started the Vitamin D and it has helped as well. I know of some who say the over-the-counter sea sickness pills can help, but I have yet to try them.

There are a couple of things I have done for the Fibro Fog that are helpful. One is to maintain a routine so that I don't lose track of keys and such.

If I have a specific place for something I use daily, I would lose track of it in a Fibro fog so I created a routine for where it is. I also make lots of lists. If there is the chance that I'm going to forget a meeting or anything else of importance I write it down on the same pad of paper and I keep the pad of paper by the phone.

I am notorious for writing lists all over the house on different pads of paper, not wanting to go into another room because I'm too busy. And then forget where I put it. Fibro has taught me to be more organized. One notebook, one place.

I do keep one in my purse as well to remember certain things. You can be as clear as day and then a Fibro fog will hit and you'll forget all those wonderful things you thought of during your clear time. FM has taught me how to reorganize and actually become more efficient. Now how's that for optimistic?

Finding time to relax and enjoy yourself is big. I kept saying it but it is important to take care of yourself. Fibro makes it mandatory. I've often wondered if this is the way the body asks you to pay attention to it. Some of the practices that help Fibro are age old remedies for peace and calm. I meditate daily without anyone around; just me and the Universe.

I have learned relaxation techniques and take a daily walk to relax. Taking time for yourself is an important part of feeling better. If you're anything like me it's hard to relax and sit back. I love to keep going and do, do, do! But Fibro has taught me not to ignore my own needs.

I haven't become a selfish witch but I have found out how to say no when needed. I have found that I don't have to fix everything. And I have found that I am not in control and that I don't need to be.

Fibro really has taught me a lot about myself. Would I go as far as saying, "Thank you, Fibromyalgia?" Hmmm.... Let me think for a... *NO!* I could have figured it out another way. But I respect Fibro for what it is. It has showed me ways to learn to take care of myself that I may have never learned before.

My family.

"Good morning. Are you feeling better?" was the way the morning usually starts. If you say "I am feeling better," then everyone relaxes and goes about eating their breakfast but if you say "I'm not quite up to par this morning," everyone feels horrible. They say, "You look so good! How can you be sick?" or "I feel just like you. I had a stiff neck as well" or "You just need to feel better!" It seems the mood of the whole household is dictated by how I feel.

I can't stand attention especially the kind that is generated by feeling 'not up to par'. I've always been that way. I love who I am and what I do. I like being appreciated as much as the next person and I don't like Fibromyalgia giving me attention.

I'd rather have my work speak for itself. It doesn't mean that your family ignores all the symptoms and acts as if nothing is wrong, but there are certain things said that don't make you feel like 'It's your fault you're not feeling better', 'You don't look sick so therefore you're not', 'Everybody as aches and pains so get over it', 'You don't have this disorder you're just have the Mulley Grubs'. That is sometimes how some of the well-meaning things that are said are taken.

How do you approach someone who lives with Fibro? Ask them if you can help them today and mean it. (And then you need to take that help gratefully instead of begrudgingly)

Look for things that may lighten their load. (You may say no, but it sure feels nice for someone to notice) Don't compare your own aches to theirs. Unless you have been in a Fibro body you really can't understand what it's like—just like we Fibros can't understand and feel what it's like to be in your body.

Don't hover and do everything for us because then that shows we are really not well. Just ask and think ahead about the things you ask us to do. Think about what it takes for us to get up from the chair.

Our feet burn, the joints ache, and the walk from the living room to the kitchen gets longer and longer. To a Fibro person who is having yet another Fibro day and is trying to conserve her energy it is a loooong walk!

Be understanding when we aren't able to vacuum or mop the floor. Any kind of repetitive movement can be murder on the shoulders, back, and neck. If there is one thing that puts me into a day of Fibro symptoms it is housework and the movement of dusting, mopping, and vacuuming.

I used to think, "I wish I didn't have to do my domestic goddess chores," but now I wish I could. Be careful what you wish for, Beth!

So hammering, mending, sewing, quilting, and housework are off the list for now. I used to be a costume designer and work 'til the wee hours designing hundreds of costumes. I loved my work.

I singlehandedly created two-hundred costumes for a production of *A Christmas Carol*. I pushed and didn't delegate any tasks to anyone else. I worked on it for two months straight and it was as if I burned myself out. My body collapsed. I only made it to one performance. I was even nominated for best costume design and couldn't make the ceremony. All because I pushed and didn't find the balance.

Fibromyalgia has reminded me about moderation and being good to myself. Sure, you can say, "But she got it done. She did it!" I used to take pride in that until I realized I was wearing out my body and not listening to what it had to say. If anything, listen. Listen to your body and make sure that others who are close to you are aware of the harder days so that they can take some of the burden off your shoulders, even if it's just to tell you they love you.

Family and friends will always say something that might come out wrong but remember where their heart is. They want you to feel well, they love you, and how they express it might come out wrong. But their heart is in the right place. They won't know how to help or treat you unless you let them know. It isn't a weakness to need some help from time to time. It is a strength to be able to ask, and it is a balance not to go overboard with what you can or can't do.

CHAPTER FOUR

No Pain No Gain — *Oh really?!*

I'm convinced that the person who said 'No pain no gain' had Fibromyalgia. Because when there is pain—Fibro pain—the by product in your body is weight gain.

Weight gain is another one of those wonderful Fibro side effects. You hurt and ache. You feel stiff from top to bottom, sometimes you can't bend from all the stiff aching joints and muscles, but you still have to eat, right? You crave carbohydrates because your body wants something to get it through the day. You're told that eating certain foods can cause your symptoms to flair but it just so happens those foods are the ones you tend to think about. You feel helpless as if the body is totally in control of you and all these feelings and symptoms make you feel even worse. You are supposed to move but you feel as if you can't. You have to move but what you are eating will keep you from losing or maintaining your weight.

Your butt seems to get more doughy and you say to yourself, "Tomorrow I will exercise!" but when you wake up you are having one of *those* days and exercise just doesn't even seem feasible. You make the quickest meals you can so that you can sit back down, exhausted. You can see how weight gain is a part of Fibromyalgia.

You'd think as strong as we all are we could overcome the cycle and just lose the weight, but Fibro has other plans.

So what have I personally done with this one? Accepted who I am physically, and just do my best from there. I used to be a size seven in my teenage years. I did five hundred sit ups a day to maintain my weight and ate whatever I wanted.

I was one of those lucky kids that, no matter what I ate, my complexion was without a pimple—and that matters when you're young. I knew that if I kept up the exercise I could more or less eat whatever I thought sounded good. When I became pregnant with my first child I craved oranges. I walked four miles every day, enjoying my pregnancy.

After giving birth it took some time to get back down to my normal size (and normal at that time was then a size nine). It was when I had my second baby that all hell broke loose. I craved carbohydrates. I sat in bed because of those 'not feeling quite right' days.

I exercised as best I could with a fourteen-month-old, and another baby on the way. I carpeted the entire downstairs of my house while being seven months pregnant. My back, neck, and spine hurt but I thought it was just from the massive baby inside.

Things changed and after having baby number two, I had an extra thirty pounds to lose. I worked at losing them but they didn't want to come off. Not two years later I was pregnant once again and was beginning to have some pretty apparent Fibro signs. This pregnancy was easier except for the constant infections and painful joints. After giving birth to a little girl I diligently exercised and tried to lose the weight. But the aching and the pain and the 'I don't care depression' started sinking in. So I fought with my body for many years (just about the weight) and then one day it hit me.

I didn't like how I looked because of what other people in normal society thought. I looked in the mirror and saw a young girl with beautiful 80's hair (back then it was beautiful) and a good mommy and wife. The weight didn't matter. As long as I exercised and did my best that was all I could do.

If I didn't worry so much about it, I reasoned, it would probably fall off much faster. And as my philosophy on life became more apparent I realized that it truly didn't matter. I was as beautiful as the next girl, just a little bigger. I began to love my body even with its extra lumps and bumps. So when I was diagnosed with Fibro and I learned that weight gain was one of the symptoms, I had already come to terms with the weight.

You don't need an excuse like "Oh, I can't lose weight. I have *Fibromyalgia*," and then turn around and eat a whole pie. You can be just like everyone on this earth who experience some kind of contrast in their lives that they may not be happy with. It's important to stay as healthy as you can, but again, there's no reason to obsess. You are who you are. You can change the weight or maybe you can't. Just be who you are and do your best.

So what do I do about my weight now? I watch what I eat and I splurge when I must. If I don't splurge the craving gets worse and then I really splurge. I exercise when my body allows me. I don't not exercise just because I feel a little tired.

I monitor where my body is for the day and then proceed with caution. I don't beat myself up over what I am eating but I do my best to keep trying. I look at myself in the mirror every morning and say something nice about my outer self that I like.

I wear clothes that make me feel good about myself and then I go out and face the world. Not another thought about weight. Being thin is not the end all be all. I learned that over my lifetime. A good attitude with an 'I'm doing my best' and truly meaning it is all that you need. Here, let me shift my doughy butt.

Aim, Shoot, and Fire!

There are some things that you want to avoid when it comes to Fibromyalgia that for some could be hard to release. I personally don't drink, but alcohol can bring on symptoms for many Fibro patients so if you can't give up your daily glass of wine maybe just cut it down a little.

I love coffee! It is the one thing I think about in the morning, and wouldn't you know it: caffeine is another no-no when it comes to Fibromyalgia. I'm not a decaf drinker. You may say it tastes just like the real stuff but it doesn't to me. Give me a Grande sugar free vanilla skinny latte any day!

What I have done is I just drink less of my magic elixir. I go with half a cup in the morning and sometimes another half in the afternoon. It hasn't affected my symptoms as of yet. Fibro knew not to mess with my coffee; that's where I draw the line!

Not sugar too!

This one is the one I can really tell. Sugar flares my Fibro like you can't believe. Sugar brings on the adrenaline and when the adrenaline leaves, here comes the Fibro flares. Again, it is next to impossible to give it all up so minute amounts are better than none at all.

I've come to the place in life that the flares are so much worse than actually eating and drinking something. I think clearly before I put something in my mouth. "Is this going to affect my whole day and tomorrow as well? Is it still worth it?"

Processed foods can also be a problem. Many Fibro patients have a chemical sensitivity to anything processed. Shooting pains become worse with any kind of sugar replacement. Hey, I tried! I've tried to replace sugar in some way but the sugar replacement affects me worse than sugar itself, so what is the lesser of the two evils?

I know it feels as if Fibro patients are sensitive to everything… Okay we are, but we do what we have to do in order to feel good, don't we?

Water is an important part of being healthy even when you don't have Fibromyalgia but if you do have Fibro, drinking water is a necessity. Water helps to replace oxygen and nutrients in your body. You need your body to be 'well oiled' and drinking water keeps you hydrated. Most people don't drink enough water. I do my best to drink at least six to ten eight ounce glasses of water daily.

Exercise C'MON!

I remembered the days of my teenage years when I felt more or less invincible. I would do five hundred sit ups a day and wonder why my neck ached. I was doing them right.

I stopped doing sit ups for a month thinking that maybe I had overdone it all the while seeing other girls and guys in P.E. surpassing the amount I could do. They weren't in any pain. They were laughing and having a good old time lifting each other up and putting each other in the trashcans. I even protected my neck through the right way to do sit ups and yet my neck felt as if it was going to fall off from the stiffness and pain. Again, another Fibro past moment I had forgotten and now realize even then Fibro was talking to me.

I had always dieted and exercised to extreme for years until I had children. I then realized how unimportant it was compared to taking care of my babies.

I walked about five minutes each day for about a week. And then something happened. I began to feel better. I didn't feel so stiff or achy so I then began walking a ten minutes. As my body got used to it I began to feel better. The symptoms didn't feel as severe and my Fibro fog seemed better.

I now walk in between one and a half to two miles a day now. If I go over that I feel that I am pushing my body. I tried for three miles and the body revolted. Don't ever push yourself but do at least get some walking in. A few minutes a day to start is worth it.

Exercise releases endorphins that release pain killers to your body. They are a natural pain reliever. I tried to add a little stair stepping and I immediately went into a Fibro flare. I thought maybe a little bit of an incline might work but alas... Fibro said no.

Stairs are a thing of the past when it comes to a department store. When I'm having a good or bad day I don't even try the stairs.

If I have a morning where I am having a hard day then I walk a little less but I do walk. It makes a huge difference in my quality of life. I used to take the stairs in any department store for extra exercise but that isn't allowed anymore. I take the escalator because the stairs put my body into a frenzy. I'm learning about what my body is asking of me and it makes life a whole lot easier. Gentle exercise is the way to go. Swimming is an excellent way to exercise as well. It is gentle on the body. Don't give up on your body and don't give up on yourself. You can do this.

A little nice refreshing walk everyday not only will help your chronic disorder but it will help your mental world as well.

Yes Doctor.
I sprained my ankle...Again!

Back in the 50's no one even acknowledged Fibromyalgia. Can you imagine how many people must have had this way back when and they were misdiagnosed? How do you put so many widespread symptoms together to create this condition that seems to affect everything that is important to living a full and rich life?

I hadn't put two and two together with all the crazy symptoms I had been experiencing since the 80's but no one would have back then. I remembered in a two year period I had been put in a cast three times because of a possible break of my ankle or foot. I would just be walking and there would be the most indescribable pain shooting through my foot.

They would x-ray it and then say it wasn't broken but thought maybe it should be cast—here we go again—just in case. This happened twice to my foot and once to my ankle.

My ankles and my feet were in pain on a daily basis and I would be on crutches more than I wouldn't but no one even suspected that this could be Fibromyalgia. I ached and was kept up at night with my feet feeling as if every bone was broken and then it began to back off and after a five year period of sprains and twists it all subsided.

How you position your feet and legs is a big deal when you have Fibro. If you stretch your toes just a little too much they freeze in position with a cramp that you wouldn't give to your worst enemy. If you lay in a certain position for too long your back freezes up and won't let go.

I'm always stretching and moving my body. There's a feeling that wells up in my body that tells me 'It's time for the shift now.' I don't wait. I listen. I listen to what it is telling me to do and when I do I am in a much better place.

My family is used to me jumping up in the middle of a conversation and saying, "Keep talking. I just need to walk around a little." And then once I stretch and move I sit back down for another twenty minutes. It works for me. Even laying on the bed during the day for too long affects the severity of pain in the joints and muscles. So the answer is to keep moving, even if it is just a little.

When did that Guinea Pig crawl under my skin?

You're having dinner and then it starts. The shaking, the tingling, the feeling as if your pet

Guinea Pig has decided to take residence under your skin. It begins in your spine and tingles up and down as your feet and hands do a little tingle dance. You feel as if there is a symphony going on in your body that makes you feel as if something is misfiring and taking you over. Welcome to Fibro Land where everything isn't as it seems.

How about we go on the Fibro rollercoaster where one minute you feel wonderful and the next minute you take a dive so deep that you wonder who made up this cruel joke of a disorder. Shall we go to the Under-the-Rib Pain Ride? Where no one can possibly explain where the pain is coming from but you know it's there no matter how much they push and prod?

Or how about the Fire Down the Spine Carousel where whatever comes around, comes around again! Who wants to take a whack at the guinea pigs under the skin? "Oh pick me, pick me! I will! I will!" Fibro Land… You gotta love it!

Yes I talk about what could be the most frustrating Fibro symptom and here is another one: The shaking, tingling, burning and tingling up the spine, the bugs under the skin, and pain under the left side of the ribs. These just seem to have no point as far as I'm concerned.

The shakes can make me feel dizzy and a little loopy in the head while feeling cold and warm at the same time. You're constantly shifting and moving in hopes something will break loose of the hold and then you just say FINE!!! I'm done! Do what you gotta do! — stopping all work and staring into space.

You can't read because your eyes are freaking out and you can't move your neck because it puts you into dizzy spells. So what do I do? I sit and meditate. I relax, sit back, and just let go. I don't focus on the pain or the room spinning. I close my eyes and just let it go.

I do know that if I am at the computer too long that it brings some of these symptoms up. It usually starts in my hands and then works its way through my whole body. I get up stiff-legged and stretch. This can help at times but mostly I just let go and realize the work will get done a little later. The evenings are my best time when Fibro doesn't seem in the foreground.

The afternoons from about three o'clock until about five o'clock are my down times. This is when I step away from the computer and kind of walk around waiting for the severity to pass which it usually does.

My body comes back to me at about five so I can get dinner done and get a little more work finished and then play some checkers with my daughter. She prefers to play checkers with me between three and five because she knows she'll always win when Mom's brain is out on a break.

Oops! Time to get up and walk... I'll be right back.

CHAPTER FIVE

Don't Take This Lying Down

You wake up in the morning and lay perfectly still. Maybe, just maybe, this will be the morning where you wake up and can get out of bed without your husband using a spatula to flip you over. You move your neck to the left and then to the right and it tells you immediately where your body is for the morning. "Honey could you get me the spatula?"

After lying in the same position you decide it's time to actually move your body. You brace yourself, wondering which part just might fall off from being stiff and sore to the very bone. You get your head off the pillow and strain your neck to sit up. "At least I got that far," you say with a dose of self encouragement. You pick up your deadweight legs that have been busy all night long bouncing to the tune *Don't Worry Be Happy* and it's now that they decide to stop.

It has left you exhausted and you haven't even gotten out of bed yet. You take leg number one and swing it over the side of the bed. You sit for a few extra moments to let your body settle in. You feel as if you've been exercising like a fiend all night long and now here are the results. But you haven't been exercising at all. Just sleeping.

You swing the other leg over and sit for a while. You finally muster up the ability to actually stand up and now it is time for the Frankenstein hobble. You walk stiff-legged, not being to bend your knees, and feel as if you've got bolts in your neck. If it wasn't so achy and stiff you'd be laughing at the absurdity.

The first thirty minutes always seem to be the worst. You put on your slip-on slippers and as you stand up and begin to shuffle, one flies off your foot. This morning you can't seem to keep them on. You feel like you're starring in a Charlie Chaplin movie. You can't bend to pick up the slipper so you kick it across the floor in hopes it lands in a place you can reach. You shuffle, kick, and then give up, taking off the other slipper as your feet plunge into the arctic cold.

Now most people can handle a little cold, but to a Fibro patient the cold is to the bone. Your feet are so sensitive that you feel as if you have stepped on ice bergs when you set them on the tile. Socks are even an issue. If they don't fit just right, they can feel as if they are cutting off your circulation. Fibromyalgia makes you sensitive to everything. You really have to think through your day and what you are around with Fibro.

If you are trying something new, a new fragrance of any sort, a new detergent or cleaning supply, you have to give it a whiff to see if it is going to affect you. I tend to get dizzy and light headed with a severe pain in my neck when something is not going to agree with me.

Yet another thing to remember in your Fibro life: Being in a room full of people with no ventilation can set Fibro off as well. All the perfumes and any kind of smell that someone might have on their clothing or body will set Fibro into motion.

When my husband and I lecture we make sure the room is easily ventilated at a certain temperature or else I will be on the floor and Lee will be picking me up with his Beth spatula. Again it comes down to listening to your body and what it needs, opposed to making it do what you want it to do.

For some time I have observed how my body reacts and what brings on a flare. Sometimes I can be doing the same routine, day after day, and still have a flare. It isn't about what is in your environment. It can be about what is around your outdoors and the weather itself. You shift and figure out what works best for you. I am at my peak in mid morning until about two o'clock when the body starts to tell on me. I do mindless easy work or just sit back and relax in the afternoon and then start back up after dinnertime.

There are a few things I have done for fatigue. Again, gentle exercise and taking the supplements helps me tremendously, but so does relaxing. Watching a funny movie or sitting around talking can keep your mind active and keep your body at rest. If my mind is up to it I take this time to do crossword puzzles. It can be hard to hold the pencil at times so I try all different kinds of positions to sit or lay down so there is no pressure on my hands or lap but I do something as I relax.

I take care not to fall asleep during the day because it will disrupt my sleep patterns for the night... Well, when I do sleep.

I use a heating pad or a scarf around my neck as well as on my back. This relieves some of the agitated tenseness as well as the ache that can accompany it. I keep it on low. Anything above that creates the superheat in my body and face and I begin stripping off pieces of clothing. In the summer days I will use an ice pack wrapped in a paper towel.

Again, being sensitive to touch, it is important to wrap the ice pack so that it doesn't directly touch your skin.

I dress in layers due to the hot cold temperature changes within my Fibro body. The winter rain makes Fibro flare and I keep the room at a certain temperature, not too hot but not too cold, fending off any kind of flare. I do know that sometimes when I am freezing cold I take a small walk.

It seems to reset my body temperature and relieves me from the cold that seems as if it came from Alaska. Do you know what I'm talking about? This isn't any ordinary cold flash in the body. It's as if everything has been frozen by Mr. Freeze and you're standing in your underwear. I've never felt anything like it even when I felt fine before FM.

I am a fan of a turtleneck since my neck seems to be a point of contention, but again, with clothing you have to find something that is comfortable. Sure, everyone wants a comfortable shirt but with Fibro patients the shirt has to be comfortable in every way. No tight neck, no tight arm cuff, stretchy so that it doesn't bind. I wear a turtleneck that isn't tight around my neck but covers the back of my neck. This keeps the neck warm where you need it but doesn't keep it warm in the front. It sounds like it is something you can just live with, the tightness or constriction but all those things can make you uncomfortable and bring on another Fibro flare.

So when you see me down the street you'll recognize me. I'll be the one in the kooky turtleneck stripping off my scarf and then putting it back on again. Just wave… I'll know you're one of the elite Fibromyalgia Club from the same scarf that you're wearing, and by the turtleneck dance you'll be performing.

When did I become a spineless jellyfish?

The back. I used to sit and wonder what I could have possibly done to injure my back so badly? The tingling and the burning hot pain up and down throughout the day. Again I realized that I had diagnosed another Fibro symptom. For our bodies to be supported our spine is surrounded by quite a few muscles that cross one another.

The muscles cross back and forth close to the spine and have neurological connections to pain centers in our brains. As a Fibro patient the pain that is processing is in overdrive. So what happens? When you move around your brain is saying, "OH MY GOD! What are you doing?! That hurts, that hurts!" Fibro brain senses more pain that is normal and that is what causes the continual back pain.

But wait...*there's more!*

The Fibro back pain can be caused by the weakened muscles that are in our backs. When you aren't able to sleep, and by having extreme and continual fatigue, the muscles become even weaker. Then you feel as if you can't hold back your shoulders or stand properly which even weakens the muscles more. So it's no wonder we experience back pain. So what can we do about it?

I've done quite a few things that have worked with total success. There are days when my back just feels weak. Those are the days I wear a lumbar support brace. You can get one from your doctor or buy one at the pharmacy. You can even get a back brace at Home Depot if you want, but they are worn on the outside of the clothes and are more snug than ones made just for the support.

The only problem with the flexible stretchy back brace is that it can feel snug and there's that constriction once again, but sometimes the weak back outweighs the constriction. You don't even have to wear it all day. I find a few hours are even helpful.

Heat works for me as well; that is, if I'm able to endure heat that day. If heat isn't any issue during the day, I climb into the Jacuzzi and turn on the jets. The warmth as well as the circulating movement helps the back. Don't get the water too warm, though, or it will set off a Fibro flare.

Lying with pillows behind my back works well. I have many small cylinder pillows that help with my lower back as well as the spot in my upper back. I just prop them up and get as comfortable as I can and relax my back.

Curling the back. I do this all throughout the day. I round my shoulders forward, tuck my lower back and butt down, and curl my center back and stretch putting my arms straight out. Then I let my stomach sag and put my shoulders back and let go, putting my arms back down. You can sit in a chair or on the bed to do this and you can also get on the floor and curling your back while being on all four limbs. The stretch feels good and stretches the back out some.

There are days when my back actually catches and I can't move it. This is when I use a very stylish walking cane and sit back and relax as much as I can. It works itself out when the Fibro loosens up.

As far back as I can remember I have not wanted neck or back massages. Someone would come at me with their therapeutic hands and I would go running. Massaging my neck sends shooting pains up and down my spine. You want my brain to scramble? Then bring me a mechanical neck vibrator. The second it begins shaking my neck I feel as if I'm going to pass out. It literally feels like my brain is shaking loose.

Can you believe what we have to do to keep these bodies in gear? I never thought I'd be thinking this much about what my body does, but it happens and I'm going to make the best of it all.

Sleep Doth Cometh.

I lay there awake again. My body is trying to rest but I have decided it doesn't know how anymore. I talk to it, I cajole it, I plead with it... What can I do for you to let me sleep? It replies in Morse code through spasms and electric tingling through my body, yet I still can't understand.

I hardly remember my dreams anymore. It's as if I am so tired my 'dream self' stopped trying, so I live vicariously through my husband's dreams. I tap him to wake him up. "Did you dream anything yet?"

He flips over and goes back to sleep. I love dreaming. I love to figure out a psychological puzzle. I sigh. Then comes the pipe organ playing in my legs and back. *Don't worry, be happy.*

I find it ironic that this seems to be the rhythm thumping through my legs. I don't worry. I focus on the happy things in life and still have Fibro. I do a body turn and the thumping stops. My tense muscles begin to relax and I drift off to be woken up once more by that song again.

There are times when the heat itself wakes me up and I rip off my socks and pull off the covers for five seconds until I get cold. I crawl out of bed for yet another pee run and then start the process over again.

My husband somehow sleeps through it all only waking up occasionally to pat me. He doesn't see my green 'envy' eyes staring at him. "I just want to sleep." If I sleep I will be more rested in the morning. If I'm more rested I'll be in a much better mood. If I'm in a much better mood everyone else will be in a better mood. And if everyone else is in a better mood, everyone is happy.

It's not like I'm a bear. I am an optimistic person. I would go as far as saying that I have a Pollyanna kind of attitude. What's wrong with being a Pollyanna? Her life was wonderful. I bet her legs sang *Don't Worry, Be Happy*, too.

If only we could get a few good nights of sleep. I've been able to do that now. I have a whole routine now that what I wrote above is now a rarity instead of an every night affair.

Baclofen has calmed the muscle spasms so that I don't wake up all night long. I have always been a light sleeper and since I started taking Baclofen it takes the edge off the pain and Lee says I don't wake up at every little noise anymore.

Creating a bedtime routine helps as well. Make sure the room is dark and quiet. If your husband snores get him some Breath Right strips and buy yourself some earplugs; just make it quiet. Turn off the computers and any kind of light so that your body and mind knows this is bedtime. Any little light can keep us Fibro folk awake since we are so sensitive to any little extra ray of sunshine.

Make sure your bed is comfortable and that you have the right kind of pillows. Just this little thing can mean a whole lot to your Fibro body. I sleep with four, yes four, big fluffy pillows and an array of small cylinder pillows. I put two big pillows under my neck, one between my knees, and one in front of my stomach to put my arm on. I place a small cylinder pillow behind my back.

This may sound like a lot but the more cushion the less chance that I will hurt from my knees bumping each other or my boobs laying hard on the bed. If I need to shift I change the whole pillow brigade. It is important to feel as comfortable as possible. I am fortunate to have a big bed so that my pillows, being the third person in the bed, have their own space too. Lee knows not to sleep with his arm on me. The pressure is too much on my body.

Go to bed at the same time each night. Establish a routine for yourself. Right before you go to bed read something light or listen to some music. Get the mind to relax and know it is time for sleep. Get your pillows all comfy and don't anticipate having a bad night. Anticipate that this could be the night that you will sleep well. Shift your focus to the good of what could happen. Don't head to bed agitated in any way.

If you watch television before sleeping find something that isn't going to leave you thinking and worried.

I can't handle an electric blanket. Too much heat and too much... *too* much! I find myself throwing my blankets on and off at night as it is. Any kind of artificial heat bothers my body. A heating pad is about as much as I can take; that, and a pair of socks. Again the Fibro body is sensitive to everything it comes in contract with.

If you do wake up in the middle of the night don't get up unless you have to go to the bathroom. Lie in bed and don't expect that you can't sleep. This is a good time to learn to clear your mind and relax. Give your mind a job.

"We're going to see how well we cannot think and focus on our body."

Begin clearing your mind and you will find a thought will do its best to distract you. Bring it back to only hearing the sounds around you and even those keep in the background. Clear mind, clear mind, retrain the mind, clear mind and before you know it you will fall asleep once again. If this doesn't work for you think of the good things in your life. No worrying aloud in the middle of the night about anything.

Make this a routine for yourself so that if and when you wake up you have given the mind something to do in a positive way. If you can't sleep why not use the time? Getting up and reading will tell your mind "It's time to get up!" and stimulate your brain so if you do need to get up, don't do it the second you can't fall asleep. Wait for twenty minutes as you clear your mind and relax.

Staying in bed and trying the retraining trick works. You'll either fall asleep from boredom or you will get the hang of thinking positive. And if you do decide to get up don't read about 'how to fall asleep'. You want your mind clear of anticipating no sleep. The key is to learn to relax your mind and body. This is an important key to helping chronic pain but we'll talk more about that later.

Make sure to get checked for any kind of sleeping disorders. Sleep apnea can be fatal and can be masking itself with your Fibro. Rule out anything that could keep you from sleeping before thinking that it's just your Fibro acting up. Anything you can do to help sleep is worth it because sleeping will help your body rest and heal, and Lord knows we need it.

I'm burning, I'm burning...
Oh wait...It's just the bleach!

There are many sensitivities that we endure as Fibro people. They might as well use us as part of the dog team on the police force. We could sniff out any kind of chemical they wanted. Of course we would have to smell the chemical first and then that would put us into a Fibro flare and they would have to wait for several days before we were up to actually being able to be well enough to sniff. Another profession down the tubes.

No one understood. I immediately would get a headache the second I had even a whiff of any kind of cleaner. I knew when Mom had gone in and cleaned the toilets because the back of my head would begin to thump and then would come the headache. I thought for sure it was poison.

As a kid I would do everything to keep from going into the bathroom on cleaning day. Then I took a whiff of onions. My eyes would water, which was pretty normal, and then I would start coughing and some of the blood vessels in my eyes would break.

The headache would come on and I knew to ask for no onions on everything. Any strong smell, but especially any kind of manmade chemicals, was a curse. If I get too close my hands begin burning and itching and I start the coughing. My usually stuffy sinuses get worse and you feel as if you can't breathe, even though you can. And if you sit around it for too long you begin a Fibro flare.

Cleaning is not worth all that! It's bad enough that our eyes burn and ache and stream from any kind of smell that might set us off. Don't forget we have super powers where all our senses have been amplified.

And are you sensitive to drafts? Drafts are the absolute worst for a Fibro patient. The draft causes all the same kind of symptoms as a chemical smell but then you add in the hot/cold temperatures involved. Like I said earlier, Fibro doesn't leave any stone unturned.

I have found a way around all the reactions to chemicals and smells for myself. I again listen to what my body wanted and needed, and through trial and error found what works for me. Maybe some of this sounds like common sense, but it took some time for me to realize that sometimes common sense doesn't come easy when it comes to the signals of your own body.

You're taught one way to be and then find out that you have to be something else with Fibro. Taking care of your body now is different than it used to be.

So I've made my peace with onions. I take a piece of bread and stick it under my tongue while chopping onions or I have someone else do the chopping. I find if I chop fast and keep them as far away from my face as possible I can tolerate them but I immediately wash my hands the second I'm done. I once forgot and when I went to rub my nose the onion smell took over and put me down for the evening. Sure, you could say I'm a big baby but I know what will cause Fibro to rear its ugly head and I'd rather keep him away. I can't eat a raw onion but I can now enjoy a cooked onion. It's all about the smell.

When it comes to smells the best thing that works for me is being in an open aired room. The smells are much more tolerable when they are only a hint than a strong odor. I stay out of the bathrooms after they have been cleaned for a good hour and I do the same when the floors get mopped.

I've been known to go out and sit on the porch for a breath of fresh air after a guest has come in with an overwhelming perfume.

We use fragrance free detergent or even something that is light smelling. I always check it at the store before I buy. This goes for any and every kind of product. I've gone through different kinds of hair dye to find a smell that doesn't overwhelm my senses. Where there is a will there is a way!

I even smell the deodorants before buying. Someone might do that just to see what it smells like but I do it to see if I can tolerate the smell *and* see if I like it. I've been known to throw out make up after buying it because the smell is too overwhelming. Most people don't think of these kinds of things but when you have Fibro flares you begin to realize how every little thing matters about feeling good.

I don't give up on smells. There are some wonderful, light, white-flowered perfumes that smell like heaven that I love to wear. I have found that I'm not able to tolerate anything with musk or patchouli.

As much as you come to recognize odors you also want good smells around. I keep light scented candles around for every room. Candles are the only odor that doesn't affect me so I indulge in having good smelling candles around all through the year. Does this sound like I'm giving you every detail of my smelly world? I just want you to know that you're not alone and that you have many options to living a life that is comfortable in an uncomfortable Fibromyalgia body.

Thar she blows!
Those Fibro Flares!

I tell myself, "I'm not overdoing it. I'm not overdoing it!" as I go about my daily routine, but if I'm telling myself that it usually means that this is exactly what I am doing. When you have Fibro, your body doesn't lie.

There is a feeling that a Fibro flare is coming and it can be headed off at the pass if you just listen to what it's saying. This usually comes about when I am exercising or making a huge meal because I'm feeling a little bit better. I have learned to adapt my daily routine in every way to make it easier on myself and my body. It is telling you something, and ignoring it will make it that much bigger. If you listen and adapt then you will find that FM symptoms won't be as severe.

It's hard to be reasonable when you're feeling like you are having or about to have a flare. Just face it. You can't be reasonable in a flare even though you insist otherwise. Ignore my body, ignore what it may say, and CHARGE! Full steam ahead! You listen to ME I say! I have found that it doesn't work. Did it ever? We may have thought it did but it didn't.

Anything—and I do mean anything—you do must be first passed through your body first. When you get up to make that big meal, think if your body is really in the position to do that. Think about all the jars you may have to open, all the vegetables you may have to cut, the lifting of the pans, the reaching for spices… Think of all of it and begin to work out a system for yourself. Maybe you have a family member who can help you with some of the steps or maybe today—just for today—it will be dinner from a box.

Children are good for wanting to help in the kitchen. Rely on any extra help you can find even though you may have been the type to do it all, you can now start a new tradition of having others help. You can actually enjoy this new change.

To most people, making dinner sounds like it's just an easy thing: throw in some ingredients and there you have it! But having FM we have to realize it isn't just that. It is about reaching, pulling, pushing, lifting, and feeling like you are injuring your body. Sometimes, if I still have it in my head to make a gourmet dinner, I do it throughout the day. Maybe in the morning I'll chop a little then later on I'll put the next ingredient in.

It may take you a little longer to get things done but do it all with ease so that you don't have the Fibro monster breathing down your back. Life changes, but you can do this. Think out your day and what you are doing. If you have a big party to go to in the evening make it easier on yourself during the day.

Rest and know not to use up that much needed energy on your daily routine. Life doesn't stop with Fibro. It just changes. Change doesn't mean that you have to give something up in your life, it just means that you have to learn how to adjust your life. If you have a problem with a way to do things that you just can't seem to do then do it in a smaller easier less body stressful way.

Rest *before* you get exhausted. Don't push yourself to exhaustion and wonder why you are feeling much worse. Listen to the body signals first and you will keep yourself from have a full blown Fibro flare.

I can usually tell if when it's time to stop and relax. My face becomes flush and red while the rest of my body stays the same. It is like my Fibro Flare alarm. "Back off now and nobody will get hurt." Now how do you do this when you're in the middle of a meeting or even standing in line at the grocery store?

I can't tell you how many times this has happened to me. I will have had an amazing morning and go to do a little quick shopping before going back to the studio. I enjoy my shopping and having a quick bite to eat and then I'll be in line and the flush face will begin. It's not like I can lie down on the floor and relax at that very moment! I realize that I have a good five minutes before I need to sit down and rest preferably away from all the lights and sounds. I find my center and drop my shoulders down into a relaxed state.

I acknowledge my body that it needs some rest and I don't dwell on what is happening in my nervous system. I breathe in deep and 'let go' with the out breath. This works like a charm for a good fifteen minutes. Once I get to the car I kick off my shoes from my burning feet and take a drink of nice cool water and continue with the same exercise of breathing in, breathing out letting my body know that you hear what it is saying and you're resting. This small exercise can keep a Fibro flare from coming on at times.

CHAPTER SIX

You Have to Think of You

When anyone has a chronic condition it can be difficult for the loved ones watching what the patient is going through, but even more difficult is being inside the body that you no longer recognize. You used to be able to work until the wee hours of the morning subsisting on coffee and a candy bar. Your mood was passionate and excited about any prospects life might bring to you and you really had the world by the tail. Then Fibromyalgia sets into your life, this unexpected permanent houseguest that needs your attention twenty-four hours a day. No longer can you push the limits and help your fellow man beyond the normal.

You have to start listening to your own body. Is this so bad? Listening to our bodies? It is when the body is doing everything it can to distract you from the life you once lived. I sometimes wonder if I had listened in the very beginning, if Fibro would have laid off. Maybe if I hadn't pushed it or just took more time off and made it easier on myself would I be dealing with such a painful, chronic condition?

I'm not sure but Fibro has taught me to listen to not only myself in general but how far I should push.

Gone is the girl who took on every task in the house as her own. "No, I don't need help! I am the end all be all woman. I'll show you. I can do it all!" Gone is the girl who would write until two in the morning and then turn around and get up at six o'clock to work even harder. "I must push the limits. I can get so much more done when I push!"

Gone is the girl who did every school and party activity for twenty-seven children all on her own. "Don't worry about it! Sure, I can whip up twenty-seven gingerbread houses on my own. I don't need anyone's help!"

Gone is the girl who took on everything to make everyone else feel more comfortable and loved. "I'll make dinner AND the five hour step cake. I love you! That's what I do!"

Gone is the girl who took on everyone else's work in the office as well as her own. "You don't understand? Here, let me help you. Oh...you still don't get it? It will probably be easier if I just do it for you. No problem!"

Gone is the girl who would push to a four mile walk twice a day instead of one. "More is better, right?! If I just push it a little more..."

Gone is the girl who needs to do it all. It is something that Fibro has given to me. Fibromyalgia has shown me it is okay to ask for help. I no longer make dinner and wash the dishes myself. I do what I can and I ask for help without guilt. I used to the feel the guilt when I couldn't do something until I realized I was taking away someone else's good feeling about helping.

Instead of staring at me like they didn't know how to keep up, they would relinquish control of duties thinking I loved doing it all when in fact I realized I didn't love doing it all. I thought it was expected of me. I thought it was a form of loving. I thought if I kept moving that I was doing all I could do to live life when in fact I really wasn't living.

Think ahead about the long run of doing something beyond what you should. Don't obsess over every little detail of Fibromyalgia wondering if you're doing something right or not. Is this going to work or not? Do what you can, do your best, and then keep living life. Fibromyalgia does not define who you are. It is just something that you have. Something that you're going to have to adjust life to but it doesn't mean you stop living.

Don't refer to yourself as the Fibromyalgia monster. Know that you have it, do what you can do to help your body adjust, and then live life. If you have to live life from your easy chair today then so be it but live. Enjoy the life that is around you. Don't sweat the small stuff when you could be enjoying what you have in your life. If the pain is first and foremost for the day, take it easy and watch a funny movie. Get your mind off of what seems to be trying to take hold of your mind by treating yourself to something.

One of my own treats is a good smelling

candle. I have a bureau full of them wrapped in plastic. When I am having a particular hard Fibro day I kick back, light one of my candles, and relax. I don't pay attention to the twitching legs because they will be there whether I say so or not, I change positions and keep relaxing. If I can't open the candle because of the Fibro hands I don't let it get me down. I ask for help and then do what I can to feel better.

Just do what you can. Don't beat yourself up over what you can't do. Even if you used to be able to do it all the time. That's done. Life is now and not in the past of 'what if and why?'

So what if I have a doughy butt? So what if I can't open the jar today. Maybe tomorrow I can walk and maybe tomorrow I can open that jar. Today I'm just going to love who I am for what I am and feel better.

Ohm –Ouch–Ohm –Ouch–Ohm

I think it's a good time to meditate. I go to my room closing the door to let everyone know it is time for some quiet time. I turn on my ethereal music and get the pillows all nice and comfy. I stretch out my back and then assume the position. Not necessarily with my legs folded up but just nice and easy. I begin. Ooooohhhhhmmmmm.

> This is nice.
> Ooooohhhhhmmmmm.
> Feeling good and relaxed.
> Ooooohhhhhmmmmm.
> Breathing in and breathing out.
> Ooooohhhhhmmmmm.
> Oh yeah… Clear mind, clear body.
> Ooooohhhhhmmmmm.
> OUCH! Stabbing pain in foot. I can do this.
> Ooooohhhhhmmmmm.
> GEEZ!!! Little gnome stabbing my toes.
> Ooooohhhhhmmmmm.
> Calming down. Ooooohhhhhmmmmm.
> Feet relaxed and legs…
> OUCH! OH MAN!

I move my foot and begin again. Here comes the fibro with its little knives for your toes. I stretch out my legs and sit in a different position. Here I go again. Relax, relax, put your shoulders down. Listen to the center. Let the thoughts and sensations just pass… Ooooohhhhhmmmmm. Sigh.

Meditation and relaxation are a lifesaver when it comes to anything in your life, but they are an absolute necessity when it comes to Fibromyalgia. When someone is in chronic pain the pain just can't be ignored. It is in the foreground, forever telling you that it is there.

Sometimes pain relievers take the edge off but most of the time you are well aware it is there. We tense our shoulders and clinch our hands struggling and fighting with the Fibro that has its grip on you. It's no wonder Fibro patients become depressed and anxious. They can no longer do what they used to be able to do. Their mind knows it and their body is letting you know things are a changing. Your world becomes smaller because you don't know what your body is going to do when you go out.

Sitting still (well, as still as a Fibro person can anyway) and learning to meditate can release some of the tenseness in your body. By meditating and learning to relax your body gets some relief. Breathing in and out and focusing on your breathing, letting everything around you just pass through the mind.

Breathe in, breathe out, let thoughts just flow but don't hold on to any of them, keep going into a deeper state of relaxation. For a while you will let the stress roll off your shoulders of not just Fibromyalgia, but everything in your life. You're giving your body a break. You giving your monkey mind chatter a rest, and you're learning a technique for relaxing.

There are many different kinds of meditation and relaxation techniques that will fit your kind of lifestyle, but I do just what I wrote above. I take fifteen minutes to a half-hour each day just to relax within, letting everything go and relaxing. If my legs act up, or my hands, I just shift and find a new position.

Don't let it distract you. See it as another one of the things that you just need to let go of during meditation. You may be doing the Ohm-Ouch in the beginning but then you will begin to find a perfect routine for you and you will be giving your physical body and mind a much needed rest.

I find meditating in the evening is the better way to go. My buddy Fibro bites worse in the mornings but as with everything with Fibromyalgia, you'll have to work out what works best for you.

There's nothing wrong with your teeth, ma'am.

I can't tell you how many times I had gone to the dentist in my twenties only to find out that nothing was wrong. I would wake my dentist up at three in the morning because the pain and aching was so intense. He would meet me at his office and do x-rays. He would then proceed to tell me that there was nothing wrong with my tooth. I had no idea what was going on. After hours of pain, it would disappear until next time.

I always seem to have a tooth problem on a weekend or in the wee hours of the morning. I had a very understanding doctor who had no idea why I was hurting but he lost many a night's sleep.

I asked him if he could just pull them.

"I can't in good conscious pull a tooth that is perfectly fine."

"Can't you just pull them all? I wouldn't mind some wooden chops."

He didn't think it was funny. Especially not at three o'clock in the morning.

It's been years since my episodes with my teeth. Any time I've had pain I just chocked it up to another phantom pain and when I finally had the two teeth in the back pulled guess what? The pain was still there. If you're experiencing the jaw and teeth problems it can be another Fibro symptom. As with everything you must check with your dentist and doctor to make sure it is from Fibro and not TMJ.

TMJ stands for temporomandibular joint disorder. The pain in my teeth always seemed associated with my ears and sinuses but now I know it is another symptom of FM.

Check for all the things that mimic the Ultimate Mimicker.

Before you begin the whole routine of taking supplements and going on a green veggie smoothie kick to treat Fibromyalgia make sure that you are checked for all the things that Fibro likes to mimic.

Check for hormonal imbalances, sleep disorders, many different conditions and diseases such as Multiple Sclerosis, Rheumatoid Arthritis and Lupus that have similarities of Fibromyalgia. And even when you have already been diagnosed with Fibro make sure you take care of other things going on in your body.

Look at it this way, if you have Fibromyalgia and you have another condition as well, the other condition could be contributing to the Fibro symptoms. If you are treated for one of the other mimickers you may be able to lessen some of the symptoms you might be experiencing.

Let's say you are in a full blown Fibro flare, the one that is like a three-year-old throwing a tantrum. You've taken everything you know and have done everything you can to feel better, but you just feel like a blob. You go into your doctor and she/he tells you that maybe there is something else going on as well.

They send you to yet another specialist and that specialist finds that you have a hormonal imbalance.

They put you on a prescription for hormonal imbalance and it helps that particular condition which also helps to relieve some of your Fibro symptoms because those certain symptoms were a cause of the hormonal imbalance.

You now have less Fibro symptoms that were really hormonal imbalance and you feel better. Less symptoms to deal with, so even if you have been diagnosed with Fibro don't rule out other medical conditions thinking that everything is Fibro related. It isn't. You still have to listen to your body and see what else it is telling you. Anything to help lessen symptoms is okay by me.

Why would I ever want to accept this Monster?

So you've been diagnosed and you are frustrated beyond belief. You can't believe that you of all people have this silly unpredictable ridiculous title that no one can pronounce condition that they won't even call a disease. You kick and scream and then just... just... WHAT NOW?!

There are only so many boxes of chocolate you can go through to numb the pain of this chronic illness. So once you get past all of that it is time to talk about the fact that you really do have something that is staring you square in the eye, daring you to do something about it. Let's start here. Accept the fact *for now*.

Accept that life is going to change some, your work style will have to change, and the emphasis has to be put on you.

I made a list of things that I felt I needed to address for myself to see how to accept and move on. Acceptance doesn't mean to roll over and play dead. It just means to accept that you have this debilitating condition and to find answers that work for you. That's all.

You don't have to kiss it on the butt and accept this purple elephant sitting in your living room. It just means to walk holding its hand until you figure out how to make him smaller in your life.

So here's my list after my diagnosis.
Am I satisfied with my diagnosis and my doctor?

I'm apprehensive about my diagnosis. I fit the profile and have been tested for everything else so yes I am satisfied. I'm not sure about my doctor yet but if I'm not comfortable then I will switch to someone who understands and supports me.

Do I feel that my doctor is there to help me through this?

They keep wanting to do one more test. I realize this is just because they want to make sure the diagnosis is correct so I am comfortable with doing more tests since I am being treated with medication and lifestyle change for Fibromyalgia.

What can I do to prevent flares?

Listen to my body and hear it when it says 'that is enough for now.' Take breaks and stretch while I'm working and begin making changes so that my body isn't stressed in everyday activities. I could give up vacuuming. It's about time someone else learned how to vacuum and do housework.

How can I get rid of some of the stresses in my life?

Paying attention to the stress in my body and not biting off more than I can chew. Not worry so much about helping everyone and let them help me without feeling as if I'm putting them out. Taking time to relax and enjoy life more as I heal.

How can I deal with these changes in a positive way?

By realizing that Fibromyalgia is just a word. It isn't a death sentence. It will help me to make some good positive choices in my life for myself that are needed right now. It will show me how to slow down and take care of me.

What things do I do that seem to make it worse?

Over exercise, over work, over…everything!

What do I have to avoid?

Working on adrenaline and coffee. Learn to live in balance instead of pushing myself until I no longer can move. Which is just what I have done. GEEZE!

What can I do if I like an activity but it makes my symptoms worse?

Try the activity on a small scale and see if it is as enjoyable. If not then go back to it when I am on the healing path and see if it is something I can do then. I can find others' activities that are just as fulfilling I'm sure.

Can I accept the fact that I don't know why this happened and it wasn't anything that I could have avoided?

Not at first but now I know that it is just something I have. I couldn't have prevented it and even if I could it wouldn't matter. I have Fibromyalgia and there is no place for blame or regret. Just moving forward to a future that will be healing.

How do I explain this to my family?

They've been waiting for answers just like me. They know I've been ill. They will be happy to know that there is finally a diagnosis and that maybe we can find the right road to recovery together now that we have a name.

After going through this list of questions I began to formulate a plan. Yes, I had FM, but there are things I could do to help keep it in the background and I accepted the fact I was going to need help and change my lifestyle for the better.

CHAPTER SEVEN

Positive Thinking

So how can positive thinking change a chronic pain illness that seems to consume your life? Realize that the Fibro monster has not taken your life away. Find what Fibro may have done for your life. Maybe you were tired of being the yes man and this has finally given you the chance to say no.

Maybe the perfectionist you once were now knows that there is no 'perfect', only what is best for each individual. Maybe it has shown you how to slow down and actually take time for yourself. Maybe it's time to find who you really are and what you are made of. Maybe…

Positive thought changed my life. It's not like I don't worry anymore but it has caused me to make a mindshift that needed to be made. Fibro helped me to become a better, more caring and understanding person. Sure, I know there could be easier ways to have done this but this is just how it happened. I no longer whine 'why me' and just take each day as it comes. I don't look to the past of why or the future of where my body will be.

It has taught me to understand that living in each moment is truly life. I have learned to look at what Fibro hasn't touched in my life and see how it has adapted my life for the better. We can ask the wish fairy to take it away or we can accept and learn from it which means it could go away. But being positive makes it better as far as I'm concerned.

Change can be scary but know that change is good. Remember that any kind of change is a chance to move forward. In the years ahead they will find either a cure or a medication that will take care of it all. Think and envision that in your future but for now live the life you have been given.

In hindsight I see what Fibromyalgia has been trying to say to me.

> "Slow down, smell the roses, don't push so hard, enjoy what you have at this very moment, relax and change your reactions to the outside world so that you feel good within. Let others help you because it not only helps you but it helps them feel useful. In this senseless illness, change is good and you'll become an even more efficient spirit full of ease and calm."

Those are just a few of the lessons I have learned. I wouldn't have known if I hadn't gotten this condition. Find the positive in the world and your environment. Something that will bring on a healthy attitude, which is something you have to have with a chronic condition.

Find humor and laugh.

This not only releases those 'feel good' hormones but it's good for your overall life. Don't just *find* humor in your day; go searching for it.

Make a date with humor through movies or even the morning comic strip. Do more smiling than frowning. It's another exercise that is important to your overall well being. Find a book of corny jokes and just laugh with milk spewing out of your nose. Release all the emotions through laughter. It works wonders on your body.

Don't become useless in your mind. Sure you have Fibro and some days you can't even remember your own name, but doggone it, you are not useless. Today your brain may be on hold but tomorrow brings a whole new day. Baby yourself on the days your mind feels slow or your body refuses to cooperate.

Scarlett O'Hara said it best: "Tomorrow is another day!" So many things can change in a day. You could get a good night's sleep, you could finally find the understanding doctor, and you could find the right medication to help you through.

Look to each day and find the joy that you can in your life. Make Fibro secondary and not the first thought on your mind. Sure, you're in pain but as you do your best to get through the Fibromyalgia maze, find what you can to enjoy—even if it is a little piece of lint your dog just brought to you.

See the love around you. Take your small walk. Enjoy your meals. Know that this too shall pass. Rely on your faith whatever that may be. We were not made to suffer here on this earth. We were meant to live and if we live in a body that doesn't want to cooperate, we listen and then still live in the best way we can. You are here for a purpose no matter what your purpose may be.

You don't even have to know it. Just know there is one and Fibro is not going to stop you from living. And as you get better and become a new and improved being because of it with new thoughts and new respect for your body and your environment don't forget to continue to take care of yourself. Don't forget the days when you felt like you do now.

Continue to respect your body and how it responds to the outside world. Take care of it understanding that you are a little different than most people. You *have* to find the balance in life because your health depends on it.

You may begin to feel like you are Superwoman but make sure to take care of yourself. You still have Fibro and Fibro doesn't answer well to, "I feel great today! I'll push it to the limits!" because that is when Fibro decides to take the driver's seat. You've been given a clear signal to begin to hear what your body is telling you and through meditation, exercise, lifestyle changes, medications, and a positive attitude you will come out on the other end of this learning much more about yourself and what it takes to feel well both inside and out.

Don't forget that you are not pain and you are not a chronic illness. You may feel limited at this very moment but you are more than just a body. You are a body, a mind, and a soul. It isn't your body who makes you, you.

It is your soul that can never be touched. It is your soul that is forever happy and healthy and that soul can override anything happening in the physical vessel we call a body. Rely on your own belief in yourself and this Universe that all the answers will be there when they are needed. In the meantime... enjoy this circus of life.

CHAPTER EIGHT

Helping Your Body and Mind

All this talk about Fibromyalgia. It makes a person want to crawl into a cave and live off the land far away from anyone and anything. Hang out with the owls and the raccoons. Who ever heard of an owl that had Fibro? Fibro Owl! Maybe we could learn something.

So now let's talk about some of the things that might help your Fibromyalgia body and mind. I'm not talking prescriptions or supplements right now I'm just talking in general that you can do at home right at this very minute to relieve some of your symptoms.

If you are dealing with Fibro fog remember that your body and nervous system are oversensitive to things around you including too much to do. Do your best to slow down and begin to focus on one thing at a time.

If you are afraid you are going to lose an important thought, then write it down but don't over stress your mind. Not only that, if you have something that requires a lot of focus, then put yourself in an environment where you can concentrate. Avoid areas full of light and noise.

The distractions may put you into more of a Fibro fog but if you are able to focus, find a place where it is less busy, and focus on one thing at a time. It will help the fog.

Find ways to adapt your daily life into an easier way of life to avoid Fibro flares. Let's say today you're going to tackle the house. Time for cleaning, mopping, and vacuuming. First, take inventory of your body and see if this is a good day. If you are in a lot of pain then hold off for another day. If you are sore and achy and think maybe a little movement is good, then do some light work but even if you are having one of the good days make sure that you figure out how to do your work a little smarter not harder.

See how you can make it easier on yourself to do all that needs to be done. Can your task be broken down into smaller steps so it isn't so hard on your body? Sometimes we don't realize just opening the bottle of cleaner can cause our hands to go into aching and pain.

I leave all the lids off my cleaning products. We don't have any small children around to worry about and it makes it easier when I do clean. I'm off limits to the mop and the vacuum so others do it for me. I had a hard time at first feeling like they were my maids but realized that if they needed me to be able to do all the other things I can do, the cleaning had to be done by someone else.

This is something I learned the hard way. You know that beautiful purse that looked wonderful hanging over your shoulder can be a culprit in starting a flare? I have been through many purses thinking maybe, just maybe, this one won't feel like an elephant on my neck and back. I've found that by just finding something small and light is the answer.

Anything that is on your shoulder whether it is a backpack or a purse can cause your Fibro neck and shoulders to stiffen and ache and this can lead to the fatigue once again. If you must carry that big bag, and you are shopping, pick up the shopping cart first and throw your bag into it to keep from carrying it. If you're at the airport use a rolling cart for all the necessities.

Don't think that because you're having a great day that carrying something, just a little, won't matter. It does. Think ahead and how your whole body is going to react.

Here's another movement we take for granted, not knowing that it can cause pain to the FM body. Think about how you move and how you handle everyday objects. We rush from the telephone to the microwave, cooking and talking, dishing up both gossip and food. But in those moments of movement that we take for granted, you just picked up the phone and moved your neck sideways to hold it along with opening the microwave with one hand and putting the plate in with the other. All these movements can cause stiffness and pain, but if you handle them just a little differently you can avoid the problem.

Hold the phone with your hand so that you neck isn't in a crazy position. Watch how you lift and multi task. Don't pick up baskets of laundry that are too heavy. Put your dishes in the cupboard at a level so you don't have to do any back bending.

Any sudden movements can all of a sudden put you into even more pain and with Fibro the pain doesn't go away. Sure, when normal people bump their arm on a chair it may hurt but then the pain goes away. With a FM person the pain creates more pain and before you know it you are flat on your back once again.

The IBS can really upset a day, can't it? You wake up feeling pretty good and then you go out the door and rush right back in to the bathroom. Sometimes it isn't about the constipation or the diarrhea it's about feeling bloated and just full of gas. You don't need me to tell you that there are certain foods that can contribute to some of the discomfort here.

Limiting your intake of certain foods can help out with the gas and bloating. I limit broccoli and beans and it keeps my bloating down to a minimum. The fiber therapy is what helps the alternating bowel movements as well as acidophilus pills. Sounds like I'm getting a bit personal? I'm just laying it out like it is. Once you've had a colonoscopy you pretty much leave the 'a bit personal' part behind... *literally.*

I'm at the computer all the time. It is what I do. I wake up and first thing I'm blogging. Then I get some morning work done before breakfast when I can get out of bed. There are a few tips to using the computer or sitting at any desk that will help the hands and your arms.

First thing I do is increase my word size in my documents. I don't want to strain because it forces me to slump and squint my eyes which both actually hurt after awhile. So, I hurt. Everybody does that but as you know the FM patients hurt beyond hurt in such a simple task. Increasing my font size keeps me from straining and slumping.

Take a lot of breaks to stretch your body. Just moving away from the repetitive movements of the computer will help your body by stretching and walking around a little.

Do your best to keep your room at a good temperature. If my hands get cold they begin to freeze up and aren't happy but when the room is at a nice temperature I'm able to work longer and with less pain.

Sit up straight. Sometimes this one can be a hard one. It's easy to slump when you're hurting and your back feels weak. If you are feeling that bad you shouldn't be sitting at your computer, you should be laying down. But if you are working and your back feels weak make sure to use a chair with good support and sit up straight and don't lean into your screen.

Some pains and aches can be relieved if you begin to recognize when you are tensing up. Sometimes I'll find that I wake up with my hands clenched or my legs tense. Start recognizing when you do this during the day and make a point to relax and loosen your muscles. Do this as often as you can throughout the day.

As you know, a smell that turns your stomach can ruin your whole day. But when you find something that smells good you want to pin it under your nose. Moodiness can be hard on you as well as your family members and there are some smells that can put you in a good mood. This is aromatherapy at its best.

Finding the smell that is just right for you is important. I prefer a Jasmine over a cinnamon smell. We are all unique in what we like and can tolerate. Find a good smell to put in your room or in your office so that you can have something that soothes you or is energizing depending on what smell it is. This can work wonders for your mind, body, and spirit.

My youngest child is notorious for coming in and asking me to help her with something right in the middle of a project and that can bring on fatigue. How's that possible? It is the interruptions when you are in the middle of something you have been focusing on.

You know when you are about to finish a project and the phone rings pulling you off track? These kinds of interruptions can throw your focus as well as tire you out. Your body shouldn't be multi-tasking and that is what happens. Ask your family to give you the space needed during those kinds of projects and don't answer the phone. It is that simple. This little tip could keep you from getting even more fatigued than you already are.

Try to keep things organized in your life. Disorganization can make your mind jump a mile a minute as well as when you completely over commit yourself to many different things. Remember to step back and listen to what your body can do. Not what it used to do but what you can do to help heal it along. Your body has been asking you to slow down and take it easy. In order to get well and stay well you have to listen to what it has to say and implement a personal plan for yourself.

The feelings associated with finding out you have a chronic illness are a combination of relief that you have finally figured out why you can't get up in the morning, to guilt and worry about how you are ever going to do this with everything that you have to do each day.

No matter how much your family tells you that they will help and do anything to get you well, you feel like it is somehow your fault that you're unable to take care of your family in the way you and they have grown accustomed.

Does this mean it's true? Absolutely not. It is all in how you handle it and how you communicate your Fibro diagnosis to your loved ones and what it means to you and their lives. Life is about change and right now your life is in a cycle of change. You can look at this change as for the better and be willing to reach out and get some help from others around you so that you can get better.

Let others know when you want help or not and don't be upset if they don't ask. They may be afraid to even bring it up, insinuating that you may be 'too weak' to do much anymore. Ask for help in a way that lets them know you are not taking advantage of them and not in a way that can be interpreted as complaining.

Don't strong arm others into feeling sorry for you, making them feel guilty if they don't help. You have been living life without asking for help up until now so it's going to take patience on your behalf and your family to understand what the new rules are in the house.

When someone asks if you need some help, answer with a kind tone whether you need help or not. Be direct and be thankful for the help you receive. Don't expect others to read your mind.

Ask, and help them understand what it feels like to have the Fibro monster. Better yet, give them something to read in order to understand you better. Others can't possibly understand how a chronic illness can hurt someone from head to toe and sometimes just giving them some material to read about the condition is enough.

To anyone who asks, "What exactly is Fibromyalgia?" I say, "It is a chronic illness that does a job on every part of your body. The aches and pain are like running a ten mile marathon without stretching. It's the feeling of being beat up and wiped out. That's what it is like."

We're a sensitive bunch, aren't we? Any amount of over 'anything' causes our bodies to go into overdrive, and every noise, light, touch, temperature, and smell seems to send us up the wall. The tingling, numbness, weakness, and burning come on in full force especially when… well… anywhere. It doesn't have to be in a room full of people or in a restaurant, it can happen when I am sitting all by myself and the body starts feeling like it was put in a blender. Shaking and tingling. There are a few things that can help these kinds of effects in your body.

I don't wear any kind of constrictive anything. On 'those' days I wear elastic pants or leggings, my sports bra, and a loose fitting dress or shirt with the most comfortable easy to pull on soft and furry boots. I make sure the clothes I pick are made out of cotton so they are soft to the skin. I don't wear any kind of fabric that can't breathe because then it makes me perspire which is an over-the-top kind of perspiration that brings on even more symptoms. So breathable fabric it is.

I wear a hat as well as sunglasses when I am outside or under any kind of lights. Avoid any kind of repetitive rubbing on any part of your hands or feet against any kind of surface. This brings on more burning and tingling.

Try not to stay in the sun too long and for that matter in the cold for too long. Again it is all about moderation and listening to your body.

Learning to listen and recognize your body's signals will help you get well.

Fibromyalgia has shown me how to live in a calmer more peaceful fashion. Even on the painful, hard-to-get-through days I now see my family as being by my side instead of someone to take care of all the time. It wasn't my duty to make sure every shoe lace was tied and every 'T' crossed. I relinquished control so that we could all live and grow through the experience. Fibro has shown me what is important in life, from the top of my aching head to the bottom of my burning feet. It has shown me how to live in quality not in quantity.

You will find in most Fibromyalgia books or web sites that taking care of yourself is a top priority both mentally and physically. You can ease your Fibro pain through the use of medications, gentle exercise, relaxation techniques, and a change of lifestyle. But you have to be willing to do all this in order to feel better.

Some decide that they will just succumb to the Fibro condition and let others take care of every little thing for them. They give up on ever having a normal life as they see it. Use Fibro as an opportunity to better yourself and your life. Don't give up. There are answers. Sure all the answers are different but they are answers. Keep trying no matter what you do. Enjoy the days where you feel great but just because you feel great. But remember… don't overdo it.

About the Author

Beth McCain is an author on Happiness, the Law of Attraction, and Living in Positive Thought. She has had Fibromyalgia for most of her life, and only recently has the medical community recognized the devastating effect it has on the patients who live with Fibromyalgia. Beth is just one of millions who live with Fibromyalgia every day of their lives, but who is determined to not allow it to affect the quality of her life. She lives in Oregon's Alsea Valley with her husband and sometime co-author, Lee McCain, and her four children.

Visit Beth at
www.bethandleemccain.com

Made in the USA
Lexington, KY
22 December 2010